# Qualitative Research in Health Care

Edited by

CHRIS BASSETT BA(HONS), RN, RNT
University of Sheffield

**W**
WHURR PUBLISHERS
LONDON AND PHILADELPHIA

© 2004 Whurr Publishers Ltd
First published 2004
by Whurr Publishers Ltd
19b Compton Terrace
London N1 2UN England and
325 Chestnut Street, Philadelphia PA 19106 USA

**British Library Cataloguing in Publication Data**

A catalogue record for this book
is available from the British Library.

ISBN 1 86156 440 6

Typeset by Adrian McLaughlin, a@microguides.net

# Contents

# Contributors

**Chris Bassett** BA(Hons), RN, RNT, lecturer in acute and critical nursing at the University of Sheffield.

**Lee Cutler** MA(Ed), PGDE, BSc(Hons), RN, nurse consultant in critical care at the Doncaster and Bassetlaw NHS Trust.

**Lorraine Ellis** PhD, BA(Hons), RN, lecturer in acute and critical nursing at the University of Sheffield.

**Mark Limb** PhD, RN, lecturer in acute and critical nursing at the University of Sheffield.

**Judy Redman** MA, BA(Hons), RN, lecturer in acute and critical nursing at the University of Sheffield.

**Louise Rigg** PhD, MSc, RGN, RSCN, research nurse at the Sheffield Children's Hospital.

**Elaine Stringer** MA(Ed), BA(Hons), RN, RM, RNT, lecturer in nursing at the University of Sheffield.

# Preface

The use of qualitative research has long been of interest to me. I suppose I must put this down to the failed experiments in British education in the teaching of arithmetic and mathematics in the '60s and '70s. In plain terms I was put off numbers and statistical analysis by the new radical teaching methods now long abandoned. Well, that's my excuse anyway. The plain fact is that I like to read about how patients react to health care treatments and how nurses and nursing affect them to the good or sometimes not so good. I like to understand what it means to be part of an experience or phenomenon; I believe that many nurses and health care workers feel that way too. That is not to say, however, that I don't understand the value and effectiveness that quantitative research can have, it's just that I find it mostly a bit boring and confusing to read. It is my experience that when proposing qualitative research to supervisors or funders of research they have sometimes stated that I should do research that is quantitative so that it can be relied upon and used to benefit patients better than the 'wishy washy' qualitative type of research. I have really had almost to beg that I be allowed to use it and have, up to now at least, found it to provide a level of real insight into health far greater than that of quantitative research. The truth is, of course, that the method used in any research should be commensurate with the question. Be it qualitative or quantitative it must match the question!

I decided that a book on the use of qualitative research was needed: there are already many books looking at the theories of research but very few that show how various research methods have been used in real-life situations. That is where this book comes in. It uses the real cases of experts in the health care research field and in my view shows what fantastic things can be found out by using qualitative research in health care. I hope you enjoy it.

CHAPTER ONE

# Qualitative research

CHRIS BASSETT

## Introduction

Current, valid and reliable research is becoming more and more important in modern health care practice. Patients' and their families' expectations are increasing, and they, quite rightly, expect their medical and nursing care to be the very best available. There is sometimes a bewildering number of research methods and approaches available to the health care researcher. This book has been written to explore the key issues related to the use of qualitative research in practice. There are many books written that systematically investigate differing types of research methodology, both qualitative and quantitative; very few, however, spend any real time considering the specific difficulties of carrying out valid qualitative research in the clinical health care setting. This book is specifically designed to help the very busy health care researcher in practice become aware of and understand the issues in undertaking qualitative research in modern health care practice and education. Real nurses who are all highly experienced in undertaking qualitative research in practice have contributed to this book. This provides a focus of practicality and, it is hoped, accessibility. Throughout the text a real attempt has been made to use clear and understandable language that is as jargon free as possible, even though this is sometimes difficult to achieve. A practical approach is used to illustrate the research, and invaluable practical advice is offered throughout each of the chapters.

## The nurse and research

Nursing research has certainly come a very long way. The role of nurses has changed hugely; they now nurse in a wide variety of environments, sometimes isolated from other colleagues, for instance when working in the community setting or as a nurse specialist, caring for patients, prescribing care and medication with a large measure of autonomy (indeed, specialization has become

1

an integral part of modern nursing). With this trend has come the absolute requirement that nursing evidence must be the best and most current available. The responsibilities of the nurse are now clear; they have changed and increased in conjunction with the expansion of the nurse's role. The patients and their families expect the nurses to have the answers and to practise in an efficient, safe and effective way. With this expectation, there is the risk that, if the nurses do not provide evidence-based care, they are increasingly likely to be called to account, either through the hospital or community trust's complaints mechanism, via the Nursing and Midwifery Council's (NMC) professional conduct committee or even through the legal system and courts.

In line with these changes, education of nurses has begun to change quite drastically. Nurse education is now fully university based and is becoming very much more rigorous in its approach to the teaching of research. A major part of the nurse's role now includes the use of evidence-based practice to underpin the care and treatment that the nurse dispenses. Over the past 30 years or so in the UK, there has been a growing effort made in nursing towards research-based practice. This has helped at least in part towards establishing nursing as a true profession. Growing professional concern with the best quality care has matched increasing governmental directives for evidence-based practice to become the norm. Research is seen by all to have become essential in improving and developing nursing care, also aiding in the evaluation of care and providing clearer guidelines for practice. This is clearly beneficial to the NHS and, of course, to the patient. The creation of up-to-date information and research can be used to change practice, enhance clinical care and assist in the essential requirement for the reorganization of care in this rapidly changing world of health care. Qualitative research and quantitative research are approaches to the understanding and enhancement of modern health care.

The next thing to help the nurse understand research application better must be an appreciation of the differences between quantitative research and qualitative research. These two similar-sounding terms describe the two overarching approaches to research. They are designed to explore two very different aspects of health care.

## Quantitative research

Quantitative research, if carried out with care and in a rigorous way, can carry with it a great deal of power. By power one really means influence. Until quite recently it has been the most dominant kind of research in health care. It is used to test out very important theories, such as the effects of new drugs and treatments on patients, often using randomized controlled trials (RCTs). Quantitative research can provide vital information relating to side effects and the effectiveness of new drugs on huge sample populations in many centres, often throughout the world:

- it features a high level of reliability (you can feel sure that its findings are dependable)
- it can be used to gather very large amounts of information into understandable forms that can then be used to enhance treatment and practice
- its findings can be tested using statistical means, helping one be sure of its reliability

## The strengths of quantitative research

The main strength of this research approach is related to its strong and rigorous scientific nature. It can sometimes provide a cogent argument for the release of large amounts of funding, often millions of pounds in the case of certain new drugs or new medical approaches. This is made possible by the rigorous nature of how the research is done. It can prove or disprove theories and is sometimes known as deductive research. This kind of research is generally considered best for those groups, such as hospital managers or the Government, who may wish to implement wide-ranging and expensive policy changes. Finally, quantitative research can be a comparatively inexpensive way of gauging mass opinion using questionnaires and market surveys.

| Quantitative research paradigm | Qualitative research paradigm |
|---|---|
| cause and effect           generalizable <br> masculine <br>                 measurement <br> statistics.         observable phenomena <br>     deduction          surveys <br>              systematic <br> mechanistic                    deterministic <br> causal relationships       hard <br>   operational definitions <br>                    hypothesis testing <br> experiment      universal laws <br>          numerical              testing <br> theory <br> positivism              reductionist <br> scientific              natural sciences <br> randomized control trial (RCT) | intuitive <br>                           subjective <br>                 interviews <br>                         inductive <br> generating theory <br>     participant observation <br> soft                      heuristic <br> hermeneutics                     pluralism <br>                     particular <br>              diaries        phenomenology <br>  interpretive      naturalistic <br> grounded theory                     journals <br>        humanistic              narratives <br> social sciences <br>              critical theory <br>                         ethnography <br> critical social theory <br>                              feminine |

**Figure 1.1** Quantitative and qualitative research paradigms.

*The weaknesses of quantitative research*

The weaknesses of this research approach relate in many ways to the way that it attempts to measure and quantify information. It uses a very rigid and systematic approach and attempts to control all of the variable factors that might influence its findings. This approach arguably makes it inappropriate to measure complex human emotions and attitudes as:

- human behaviour is wholly unpredictable
- nursing care does not lend itself to RCTs, as it is humanistic and individualized
- quantitative research tends to present its findings in ways that have little meaning for nurses

## Qualitative research

Qualitative research in a way is the opposite of quantitative research. It is very different from RCT for instance; the research is much more orientated to understanding human nature, and as such the researchers get close to the research subjects. This is its main strength: by using this kind of research you can understand how nursing or health care really can affect the patient. It can provide vital information on attitudes and satisfaction, and this kind of information can then be used to improve care. Research methods that use this approach include action research, grounded theory, focus groups and phenomenology. These and other types of research approach findings from qualitative research can sometimes be taken on and used to base quantitative research studies on later.

*The weaknesses of qualitative research*

The main criticisms that are often levelled at qualitative research are those that relate to its perceived non-scientific approach. This usually comes from those who are used to using only quantitative research. However, in order to produce good qualitative research a clear and rigorous research method is also needed. Other weaknesses include:

- it can be comparatively expensive to carry out as it often relies on one-to-one interviews
- the sample sizes are much smaller than the other types of research, sometimes only five or six participants

## Conclusion

Generally speaking, the two types of research approach do not work together well; however, some of the more recent studies carried out into health care have successfully adopted the two approaches to look at certain problems from two view points. This is increasingly the case. This can be particularly useful when one considers the ways that nurses need to change care. The qualitative research will explore the patient's views on a particular approach to treatment, whereas the quantitative research will provide managers with vital and dependable information that might enable them to put real money into a project. In reality, of course, in order that nurses can make the innovations in practice so necessary, they need to be aware of and use both approaches to enhance the care that they provide.

## Qualitative approaches to research

Qualitative approaches to research have their origins in the field of social anthropology and sociology and are associated with the social sciences.

- Qualitative research is usually adopted when little is known on a given topic and is associated with inductive forms of reasoning in an attempt to generate theory.
- This type of research stresses the socially constructed nature of reality, the intimate relationship between the researcher and what is studied, and the situational constraints that shape inquiry.
- This research is usually undertaken in a naturalistic setting where events are normally allowed to take their course unaffected by the research.

The context of the research is recognized as an integral part of the phenomenon or topic under investigation and described in considerable detail. Qualitative research centres on the study of individuals and/or groups of individuals in an attempt to capture their perspective and meanings. Accordingly, all types of sampling in qualitative research are purposive. The researcher aims to make explicit the knowledge, meanings and perspectives known implicitly by those within a particular society. Thus, qualitative researchers seek answers to questions that stress how experience is created and given meaning.

Several research designs or strategies fall under the heading 'qualitative research', and the most commonly used of these approaches are discussed in the following chapters. I hope you find them interesting and lead you to a better understanding of their uses, and – who knows? – may even lead you to use them to find out more about patient care.

# CHAPTER TWO

# Focus groups

ELAINE STRINGER

## Introduction

Much has been written about focus groups in recent times. They are widely used for market research and political decision-making and, as a result, have gained a negative reputation within academic circles. They are, however, a potent means for collecting qualitative data on health-related subjects, which are concerned with perceptions, values and beliefs as opposed to numerical evaluation.

In this chapter I will demonstrate the effectiveness of focus groups through reference to studies I have undertaken or supported at masters level. I will begin by giving an overview of a study I undertook. Further to this I aim to explore my reasons for using focus groups and reflect upon the principles that influenced my management of the research process and data analysis. In addition, I will consider the difficulties, real and potential, that I encountered.

## Background to study

I managed and delivered a six-month, clinically based course for post-registration students. The students attended on a part-time basis, and the course consisted of 30 taught days at the university and 30 days of supervised practice within the clinical environment. The taught aspect of the course had a rigorous evaluation strategy, which enabled the effective development of the course to meet the students' differing needs and developments in specialist fields of practice. By contrast the clinical placement evaluation was based upon verbal feedback sessions and the placement educational audit. Through these discussions it became apparent that there were wide variations in the quality and nature of supervision. However, the audits did not clarify the situation. They provided me with some information, for example the number of supervisors, their specialist qualifications and learning resources, but they did not tell me what actually happened during supervised practice.

It could be argued that the multiple variables – for example different placements, the past experiences of the student, differing supervisors' abilities – prohibit a holistic and definitive opinion regarding supervised practice. However, there is a statutory obligation for all students to be supervised by an appropriately qualified nurse. This nurse should hold other professional and academic qualifications and have relevant experience in that field of nursing practice. The role of the supervisor is to oversee the activities of the student, assess the student's competence to practise and sign the appropriate documentation to verify competence. Clearly the role of the supervisor is integral to any course. While reflecting upon the feedback sessions, I became increasingly aware that I made assumptions about supervisory practice based upon my experience of being a supervisor. In reality I had very little knowledge about how supervisors and supervisees interpreted this situation.

## Defining the question

Although I had identified a problem, defining the question took much longer. Getting the question right is an important consideration. It is the question that drives the research! The adage 'garbage in, garbage out' in computer usage can be transferred to the research process. If you do not know what you are asking, how do you know whether you have got an appropriate answer? Having a hunch is not the same as having the essence of your idea written as a research question. While ineffective research may be an academic setback for you, it should be remembered that participants in your research take part in good faith, often assisting you in addition to their own work. They expect the research to be conducted thoroughly and professionally and for their efforts to be relevant and valued.

It took me many frustrating meetings with long-suffering colleagues and my supervisor before I decided upon 'Supervised practice – what does it mean to supervisors and supervisees?' The emphasis was very much upon the individual's beliefs and their values regarding supervision. However, even at this stage I was unsure as to whether I would need to undertake a study or merely apply existing research to my situation.

In order to inform myself, I conducted a literature review. I used multiple sources of information, which included local and national libraries, organizations and relevant computerized information services. In addition, I had the opportunity to discuss my research with several colleagues who had conducted similar or related studies. Through my efforts I concluded that most of the writings were anecdotal as opposed to research based. This in itself was very interesting! Supervision is generally accepted as good practice, and yet there is a dearth of empirical evidence to support this activity.

## The literature review

I found the literature review interesting, frustrating and also comforting because I realized I was not alone with this difficulty. It also helped me to clarify my thoughts and clearly focus upon the topic. I was able to develop a conceptual framework through which I could define the key concepts and also their inter-relationships. It was also addictive because I was always looking for that last piece of research that would give me the answer. Eventually, I realized that the research was not there! I needed to discover the answer to my question.

## Research design

The problem, the question and the lack of empirical evidence all compounded my belief that I needed to conduct a qualitative piece of research. This was completely at variance to my original plan, which was to undertake a quantitative approach using a structured questionnaire. This change evolved through the process of reasoning, arguing and investigation. The lesson I learnt from this was that you have to have an open mind, consider different aspects, challenge your ideas and be prepared to make major changes if you are going to answer the question you posed.

The strengths of qualitative research are that it allowed me to gain an inside view of other people's unique experiences and recognize the multiple realities that exist for the individual group members. However, I also had to consider the impact of the weaknesses upon the study. A criticism of qualitative research is the lack of validity and reliability. I recognize this criticism; however, I agree with Lincoln and Guba, cited in Marshall and Rossman (1999), that validity is inappropriate to qualitative research. The central issue is that of trustworthiness. The study should be credible, transferable, consistent and confirmable. My aim was for procedural objectivity, which required me to declare any bias and prevent it from contaminating the evidence and faithfully represent the participants' views. My concerns were that this study was procedurally sound and I provided an identifiable path of investigation.

There are several approaches to qualitative research; the one that appeared most appropriate to my research question was that of ethnography.

Definitions of ethnography focus upon the importance of the culture. The phenomena to be explored need to be within the natural setting because human activity is based upon social beliefs, values and understanding. Cultures are dynamic, flexible and evolving; therefore, ethnographic studies are not concerned with making generalizations but with understanding a specific situation. In my study, I felt I could not view supervision within the context in which people were supervised. The literature review clearly showed the demands of the clinical environment impacted upon the type and quality of supervision.

## Ethical implications

I was acutely aware that using a qualitative approach had ethical implications for the participants of the study. Asking people to expose their feelings and beliefs may leave them in a vulnerable position. It is important to consider the ethics of any study and balance protecting rights, privacy and confidentiality while obtaining data. The way I chose to address the issue was to use informed consent. I appreciated that giving the information about the study may have the potential to influence the participants' responses. However, I considered an open and honest approach to be ethically and morally appropriate.

To promote informed consent I gave all the participants a detailed information sheet (see Appendix 1 at the end of this chapter), which identified the boundaries of the study and the role of the researcher, prior to attending the focus group. I requested that they read and complete a consent form (see Appendix 2 at the end of this chapter) before the study commenced, and during the study I had an independent researcher monitor my activities. All participants were also given the opportunity to read and request changes to the transcript before analysis. In addition to addressing any ethical implications, this had the effect of emphasizing the formal nature of the study.

This was an important consideration for me because there was the inherent risk of researcher bias. I was undertaking research in an area where I work and where I am well known by supervisees and supervisors. Morse (1989) advocates the use of consent forms in this situation to prevent situations arising where the participants treat the researcher as a consultant/colleague or friend and to create boundaries to work within. This is an ongoing consideration for many nurse researchers who are conducting studies within their own clinical environment. The advantages are that the nurse has a good understanding of the environment. Furthermore, people are motivated to volunteer for studies, conducted by a colleague, where the question arises from practice. The disadvantages are that this relationship may affect the validity of the results. Ensuring the study is rigorous and objective is an important aspect of the researcher's role. The findings should present the reality as opposed to providing preferred answers. A further consideration was that of confidentiality. Outside of the group, access was restricted to my supervisor, the independent researcher and myself. I was concerned that no harm should arise from this study. Consequently, I prevented the identification of areas and individuals and destroyed the data after the conclusion of the study.

In the account so far I have endeavoured to give some insight into the decisions I took when planning this study. That is not to say that this is the best or only approach. I chose to undertake the study in this way because I felt that it would give me the information I needed, my methods could be audited and it was ethically and morally appropriate. When conducting a study, it is easy to become absorbed in the subject and the quest for data. What you need to keep in mind is 'what data and at what cost to the individual'. While the goal may be an in-depth understanding, it should not be 'at all costs'. Consequently, you need to consider how you will collect the data in a way that is appropriate to the question, and in an effective and efficient manner. I chose to use focus groups, and the rest of this chapter will concentrate upon this aspect of the study.

## What are focus groups?

Focus groups are a means of gaining a large amount of data within a short time span through the spontaneous exchange of ideas between group members (Morgan 1997, Sloan 1998). Indeed, the focus group is reliant upon the verbalizing and sharing of ideas. It is this exchanging of views that stimulates deeper thinking around the subject. A focus group, although an informal technique for gaining data, is well planned and organized. Ideas about assembling a group of people for a 'chat' are totally erroneous.

Focus groups can be used in a variety of ways. Morgan (1997) identifies that they can be used in combination with other methods, for instance observation or interviews. Here the purpose is to generate ideas for further investigation (Greenbaum 1998) or explain data obtained through another methodology. There is a general belief that focus groups need to be used in association with other methods; however, Morgan (1997) comments that they can produce sufficient data when used as a single methodology. For the purpose of this study I chose to use focus groups as a single methodology, mainly due to time and financial constraints. I am aware that there are arguments against the use of a single-method study, and I appreciate that a combination of methods may have provided a more holistic picture.

Morse (1989) proffers the notion that pragmatic validity is increased by the use of multiple sources of data collection. This is supported by the work of Proctor (1998), who comments that validity is increased if a triangulation of methods is used. However, there are disadvantages to the use of triangulation. Proctor (1998) is of the opinion that the study time is lengthened and that the researcher must be equally skilled in qualitative and quantitative research techniques. There are also the dangers of the focus of the study being lost and the fact that different methods may not produce corroborative data.

The main advantage of using focus groups is the richness of the data expressed by the participants. The group promotes interaction and also inhibits individuals from giving misleading information (Sloan 1998). Participants are able to qualify their statements and the researcher can explore the responses (Stewart and Shamdasani 1990). In addition, Stewart and Shamdasani (1990) and Morgan (1997) comment that it is quick, flexible, cost-effective and relatively easy to arrange.

The criticisms of this method are concerned with the effect of group dynamics. Stewart and Shamdasani (1990) identify difficulties arising from dominant members who may lead to the exclusion or intimidation of quieter group members. Morgan (1997) comments that there is a risk of the participants polarizing the group. Either effect may result in individuals proffering views that do not reflect their true opinion. In addition, participants may be reluctant to divulge issues that are sensitive for them or may give edited versions of events.

I chose to use focus groups after consideration of other possible methods, namely observation and interviews. In comparison with individual interviews it is recognized by Morgan (1997) that focus groups give a broader view as opposed to an in-depth interview. However, he also recognizes that the depth of the information is dependent upon the subject's willingness and ability to talk about the topic on an individual basis. While it is recognized that focus groups may be a quick and efficient means of collecting data, Morgan is aware that there may be difficulties in assembling six to eight individuals for each session. In contrast, it may be easier to arrange individual interviews; however, the time involved in the process of interviewing and analysing the data per interview may be far greater than that needed for a focus group (Morgan 1997).

Observation, as a research methodology, offers the advantage of gaining data in the natural setting. Conducting focus groups is recognized as being divorced from practice (Morgan 1997); consequently, the emotional context of the environment may be lost. Observation also allows for the recording of a diverse range of interactions, whereas focus groups rely predominately upon verbal explanations of behaviour (Morgan 1997). However, I was concerned regarding the practical difficulties of observing practice in a variety of clinical areas and Trust hospitals. As a part-time researcher working on my own, this would have been too time-consuming and expensive. In addition, I was aware of the risk of behaviour change as a result of being observed.

Reviewing these advantages and disadvantages of using a focus group influenced me in my preparations. The old adage 'forewarned is fore-armed' was certainly applicable to me. I endeavoured to try and address each and every issue beforehand and made contingences for all foreseeable events. On reflection, I would not repeat this: it was extremely time-consuming and stressful for myself. Furthermore, most of my efforts were not needed!

As a researcher, you need to consider how to manage the focus group to best effect. This includes clearly identifying the sample group and considering how you are going to approach them and recruit them to your study.

## Sampling strategy

The key principles that underpinned my recruitment strategy were appropriateness and adequacy (Morse and Field 1996). Appropriateness is concerned with choosing participants who have the relevant knowledge and experience to inform the study. Morgan (1998b) refers to this practice as purposeful sampling, in that the participant is able to answer the research question and that the appropriate composition of the focus group will result in good discussion. This was important for me. I needed people with relevant current experience to give me their views. Initially, I considered a mixed group of supervisors and supervisees; however, I later thought that this mixture of people of different grades, power and position could inhibit the discussion. Consequently, I organized separate groups of supervisors and supervisees in an effort to make the participants feel comfortable with each other. Greenbaum (1998) supports this notion by stating that the participants should share similar backgrounds, experiences or status to enable a good exchange of ideas. Morgan (1998b) stresses the need for the group to feel comfortable. When they are comfortable, they spend less time exploring personal background and gaining trust and are more willing to self-disclose, and consequently more time is devoted to discussing the research topic. The supervisees' group consisted of six students who worked at a variety of hospitals and had attended the course, together, for three months. The group of seven supervisors all worked in the same Trust and knew each other. I found this division of groups to be effective. The groups interacted well and produced a large amount of relevant data.

I recognize the disadvantages of recruiting acquaintances, for example the unspoken agreements not to discuss certain topics or assumptions of knowledge, which may exist. Morgan and Krueger (1993) are of the opinion that, while it is generally accepted that strangers should be recruited, in reality this is not often the case. Indeed, they state that in many instances this is unavoidable if one considers the logistics and cost of assembling strangers with similar backgrounds. Certainly this was my experience. In the time I had available and with limited funds, I was unable to recruit from other areas of the country. I think the key issue is to realize that this may influence how people respond and try to minimize the impact by fully informing the participants of the aim of the study at the time of recruitment. In addition, it should be remembered that, when collecting data, non-verbal communications and their impact are recorded as data.

The second principle, put forward by Morse and Field (1996), is that of adequacy. Their interpretation of adequacy is that sufficient, relevant data should be generated through the participants. Consequently, the number of participants is important. Hague and Jackson (1987) suggest that, if focus groups are to be used as a single methodology, the minimum number of participants should be four, with a preferred number of eight to ten members. The aim is to generate discussion while at the same time allowing everybody to participate.

The number of focus groups is dependent upon the data received. Morse and Field (1996) state that there should be sufficient to give a good depth of vision of the phenomenon until saturation point. Morgan (1998a) recognizes that, if only one group is used, the information may be unique to that group and not give a clear view of the phenomenon. A greater understanding is gained through using a multigroup approach, which enables the researcher to compare and contrast the findings. Greenbaum (1998) comments that the factors which determine the number of the focus groups are, in reality, the budget and time available. In the small studies that I have conducted and supported, we have gained sufficient information with two different groups of six to nine participants, per study, to answer our research questions.

The recruitment of a suitable sample for my study was heavily influenced by the work of Morgan (1998b). He emphasizes the need for careful planning if the objectives of the focus group and ultimately the study are to be achieved. This supports the work of Morse and Field (1996), who comment that recruitment is a crucial aspect in the preparation because the participants are central to the study. Initially, I was advised to place a poster, giving details of the study, in several prominent sites in the clinical area. The aim was to inform people of the study without directly asking them to participate, which removes any threat of coercion. While I appreciate this sentiment, I was reluctant to use this method. My main concern was that, like many other posters, it would be ignored. In addition, although I had access to a 'desk-top publishing package', for a really effective poster I felt I would have needed professional assistance. Unfortunately, I did not have an advertising budget! Consequently, I informed potential participants verbally and asked those who were interested to contact me. Those that did received an informative letter and a consent form. All participants were sent reminder letters clearly stating the venue, date and time one week prior to the focus group. Again, this needs to be planned and you need to keep records of all this documentation.

Morgan (1998b) provides a checklist for successful recruitment. First of all, the researcher should demonstrate the value of the study to the participant. I discussed, with the participants, the altruistic nature of this study, namely that future supervisors and supervisees will benefit from their input. Unlike market research groups, I was unable to provide monetary incentives. In addition, I would be concerned regarding this influence upon this research. Secondly, the researcher should make personal contact with the individuals and build upon existing relationships. I personally discussed the study with all the proposed participants, and I was well known to them. In this way I was able to build upon existing relationships. Personal contact is an important aspect of recruitment. Recognizing that people have volunteered and then providing them with frequent relevant information involves them in the research process. From a researcher's point of view, this can be a time-consuming exercise, particularly when you are trying to meet with people in the clinical area. Often workload demands dominate and any meetings you arranged are marginalized, shortened and often cancelled.

## Selection criteria

Identifying appropriate criteria for selection was another issue to consider in the preparation period. Morgan (1998a) comments that a screening process should be employed. This was a relatively easy process in that I defined two groups, one group consisted of qualified nurses who had supervised students within the last three years. The second group was limited to students who were currently undertaking one post-registration course. Originally, it was planned to recruit from a larger group of past and present students, working within a variety of Trust hospitals. Owing to difficulties gaining the agreement of several different Ethical Committees in different Trust hospitals, this approach was not possible within the allocated timeframe. Although my study was somewhat curtailed by this, I did learn an enormous amount from discussing my study with a representative of the Ethics Committee, and I would advise anyone interested in conducting research to make contact with this department at an early stage in their planning. As a part-time researcher, the practical realities of accessing participants and meeting the requirements of the different organizations can and do limit the study.

## Initial problems encountered with focus groups

Hague and Jackson (1987) stress the need to make the timing and venue convenient for the participants. This was negotiated with both groups; consequently, the supervisees met in the education centre, while the supervisors chose to meet in the hospital setting. Originally, they wanted to meet in the ward area. However, it was felt that there could be too many distractions, that it would be difficult to maintain confidentiality and that the open area may impair the recording. In the end, we met in a teaching room within the hospital. On reflection, this was not a good area, because the participants were unable to divorce themselves from the demands of the clinical area. Although we were not interrupted, a feeling of tension prevailed and I was concerned that I was interrupting a busy day and adding to their workload.

We met at lunchtime, and, while this was generally accepted as a convenient time when participants can refresh themselves, it did present some problems. I had allocated one hour for the focus group, but it actually took two hours. This was because only one person arrived punctually – the others had to remain in the clinical area for a variety of credible reasons – while the rest of the group actually gathered over a period of three-quarters of an hour. This left some of the early arrivals feeling guilty at taking an extended lunch break and the late arrivals feeling apologetic and anxious about meeting their afternoon commitments. I was concerned that if the session was cancelled I would have difficulties rescheduling the group and I might face a similar or worse situation. The group preferred to stay, and the discussion eventually started an hour late.

A further problem was that the discussion was being taped and people were trying to contribute while at the same time competing with the sounds of eating. As a consequence, I felt very agitated during this session. I was concerned that the issues would not be fully explored and was aware that the dialogue was not as fluent as with the student group. My response was to move from being a low moderator to a high moderator to make the most effective use of the time.

By contrast, the students' session was undertaken in a university classroom. They all arrived on time and fully participated in the discussion. This was seen as part of their school day, they were untroubled by the demands of work and I provided hot drinks and biscuits to produce a convivial atmosphere.

## Preparation of the moderator

The group has to have a well-defined purpose and the researcher provides the agenda and guides the group to ensure that the objectives are achieved (Stewart and Shamdasani 1990, Morgan 1998a). Some authors (Stewart and Shamdasani 1990, Morgan 1998b) comment upon the importance of the researcher's balancing the need to achieve the objectives with the need of the group to express what is important to them. Krueger (1998), Greenbaum (1998) and Morgan (1998a) stress the importance of the researcher being well prepared. This involves creating an environment conducive to discussion, developing an appropriate agenda and organizing an efficient and effective means of data collection. The researcher needs to listen keenly to the discussion and act to explore and clarify issues at the same time as being aware of the personal and emotional context.

When preparing the written guide (see Appendix 4 at the end of this chapter) for the participants, the researcher needs to consider whether they wish to assume a low- or high-moderator role when managing the focus group (Morgan 1997). A low-moderator role involves introducing two or three broadly stated topics and providing neutral questions to generate ideas to gain an appreciation of what the experience meant for the individual. This is the approach that I adopted for this study, and it worked very well for the students' focus group. However, I had to change this approach to effectively moderate the group of supervisors who needed more structure to the session. With this group I assumed the high-moderator role, which is more directive, the questions are more structured and a larger number of specific topics are discussed. Stewart and Shamdasani (1990) comment that the latter approach is more likely to be influenced by the moderator's beliefs or values. This is because the participants respond to specific questions as opposed to spontaneously introducing relevant information. Instead of asking questions, I repeated their phrases, used non-verbal prompting and asked them to explain aspects more fully. The difference in the two groups was stark: the students were very verbal by comparison and appeared to have a more open response to the group, while the supervisors were more reticent, but this may have reflected their response to the workload demands that impinged upon their group. From a researcher's point of view, I found the high-moderator role quite stressful and was very sensitive to the fact that my interference may have directed the group's responses.

The moderator aims to gain good group interaction, which involves all the participants (Morgan 1997). To do this they must employ good interviewing techniques (Stewart and Shamdasani 1990) and also prepare a non-threatening environment, conducive to the discussion (Krueger 1998). Morgan (1997) and Stewart and Shamdasani (1990) recommend a circular seating arrangement. I have used this in all the focus groups I have managed and have found it to have always been effective. This allows for good eye contact, gives sufficient personal space and facilitates the audio recording. To prevent distractions during the discussion all audio equipment must have been assessed as fully functional prior to the session. This was particularly pertinent to a study when I acted as an independent researcher. The machine was fully operational before the focus group commenced; however, at the end of the session, the researcher discovered that it had not worked and none of the discussion had been recorded. This was a huge personal setback for the researcher who had to repeat the activity, with a different group, which caused a lengthy extension to the study. In addition, she felt that it was a huge loss to her study because the discussion had been so productive and yet she had no hard evidence for analysis.

After the focus group, the tape needs to be transcribed and several copies made of the transcript to enable analysis. Depending upon your computer skills and the clarity of the tape, this can be an extremely time-consuming activity. Always keep an original for reference because the other copies may be dissected during analysis and in doing so you may divorce the statements from the context, which could result in a misrepresentation of the data. Any copy of the tape or transcript must be locked away in a secure place to ensure confidentiality, and upon the conclusion of the study the tapes and transcripts must be destroyed.

## Managing the focus group

It is essential to prepare the room before the participants arrive. You should know the number of people involved and ensure that the room is of an appropriate size and furnished with sufficient chairs, a table and any recording equipment you will need. Where possible, the room should be in a quiet area and signs positioned to inform others that the focus group will be taking place and that they should not interrupt.

The chairs should be positioned around the table. This will enable the participants to face each other. It is anticipated that this will promote inclusion and discussion and allow for all comments to be recorded. The audio recorder should be placed in the centre of the table where it is visible to the participants and where the researcher can easily check that it is working.

I also found that, initially, the participants were a little nervous of being taped and on occasions had to be reminded to lean forward when they were speaking.

Behind my seat I had placed four flip charts, each with a topic for discussion clearly stated. I did this to focus their attention on the subject, but also I tried not to ask direct questions so I was able to point to the word and open the discussion by stating 'I would like you to discuss supervision', and at preset times I was able to direct their attention to other issues in the same way. I also used the flip charts as a means of summarizing what had been said.

When the participants arrived, I greeted them by name and offered refreshments. My aim was to create an environment conducive to discussion. For the students, I wanted to make the distinction between the focus group activity and their usual classroom setting. For the supervisors, I was recognizing that they were forfeiting their lunch break and also attempting to accelerate the proceedings.

Where possible, start on time; of course, this is dependent upon the participants' punctuality; however, if you do allocate time for refreshments at the beginning, it does allow late arrivals to cause minimal disruption to your session. Again, you have to consider that the participants may be doing this in addition to their usual work and they have other demands on their time. While this may be all-encompassing and important to you, they may see it as another task to be got through.

Begin the session by reiterating the reason for the focus group. You may refer to the letters you have sent out, but it is also useful to have a list of key points you wish to state before the start of the session (see Appendices 3 and 4 at the end of this chapter). These are essentially the ground rules and should include the aim of the focus group, the need for and maintenance of confidentiality, how the data are to be collected, access to the data, use of the tape recorder and why there is an independent researcher. You should clearly state that if any participant does not agree with any of these aspects they are free to leave and that their withdrawal will in no way influence your relationship with them as a colleague or teacher.

At this point, it is worth asking all the participants to speak into the microphone to ensure that the equipment is working properly and to remove any concerns regarding being recorded. Once the discussion has started, the researcher's main roles are to maintain the momentum of the discussion and to ensure that the issues are addressed. At the same time you need to resist the temptation to ask directive questions but instead let the discussion evolve. It can be a little disheartening when the speech is sporadic and when there appears to be an endless silence. In reality, the silence is usually quite short and the group will recommence discussion without any intervention. However, you need to listen intently and be prepared to rephrase or repeat a previous comment to promote further discussion.

During the focus group I used Post-its to jot down ideas as the participants said them. I used different coloured ones for the different aspects we discussed. For example when discussing perceptions of supervision the key areas identified on the flip charts were: 'supervision', 'preparation', 'influencing factors' and 'anything I have missed'. At the end of the discussion while the participants were having refreshments, I quickly stuck the Post-its to the relevant flip chart. I was then able to summarize the discussion by referring to their comments and was also able to group certain elements together. This enabled me to undertake some intuitive analysis and also supported the taped dialogue and acted as an additional reference during the analysis.

At the end of the session, I thanked all of the participants and also informed them that I would make the transcripts available to them for comment and possibly amendment before I started my analysis. I did this within a very short period of time while the experience was still fresh in their minds. However, I noted that nobody questioned the content or asked me to make any changes. Possibly the 40 pages of single-spaced text deterred them (it is better to be concise).

After the focus group, it is important to collate and identify the data as soon as possible. It is important that any labelling you used is in code form and that the data are stored in a secure area. After this, relax! You will find that while the process has been exhilarating, challenging and even fulfilling the intensity of it can be exhausting.

## Analysis

Analysis, like all other aspects of the research process is dependent upon the question you originally posed, did you intend to describe or interpret what was happening? This serious issue is supported by Burnard (1998), who clearly makes the distinction between 'seeking information' and 'seeking to understand'. The aim of my work was to describe what happens during supervised practice and compare the findings with the existing literature. The importance of this distinction is that, in describing it, the researcher is voicing the participant's perspective. In explaining, the researcher is aiming to interpret that viewpoint, to make sense of the data.

Krueger (1998) uses the analogy of the detective story when describing the process of analysis. I would agree with this: you are examining the transcripts for clues and links to commonly expressed viewpoints. Just like in the best detective stories, you may follow false leads or in other instances you will suddenly realize the intention behind what somebody has said.

This challenges your previous assumptions and causes you to reflect on the context and associated non-verbal communication. Your emotions range from boredom and the 'getting through it feeling' through to the excitement of sudden insight.

The immersion and editing styles of analysis interested me. Immersion analysis refers to the 'intuitive crystallisation of the data' (Polit and Hungler 1997). Owing to my inexperience as a researcher, I lacked the confidence to use this style. However, it did appeal to me, and, while I was managing the focus groups and during the early stages of analysis, several issues were obvious, which I was able to identify and confirm during my summary of the sessions. The editing style involves reviewing the transcripts and identifying themes, categories and concepts, trends and patterns (Morse and Field 1996). I chose this approach because it gave structure to my analysis, which came from the data as opposed to preconceived ideas (see Appendix 5).

There are several difficulties inherent in the analysis of narrative data. The volume of work can be excessive (Polit and Hungler 1997), particularly when the responses are long or unfocused. In addition, there is the complexity of the text. Unfortunately, people do not talk of one aspect at one time but instead draw on past experiences or introduce new and other possibly related issues into their conversation. You also need to consider the language that is used and how it is used. Cavanagh (1998) remarks upon the danger, when categorizing text, in assuming that similar words and phrases hold the same meaning – very often they do not. During analysis, you realize that certain words or phrases are used repeatedly but in different contexts and you wonder why you did not notice or clarify this at the time.

Through repeated readings of the transcripts and listening to the tape, I became familiar with the content and was able to identify themes, similarities and differences (Burnard 1991). I gained an understanding of the data (Morse and Field 1996) and a feel for what was being said; indeed, by the end of the analysis, I had almost a word-perfect recollection of the transcript. I was aware that the research question should dictate the analysis (Stewart and Shamdasani 1990) and also that I was responsible for deciding the relevance and, therefore, the inclusion of comments. Although I was reluctant to label sections as 'dross' (Morse and Field 1996), I did remove some of the text that strayed from the focus of the study. However, all data that were excluded were referenced, retained and reviewed at intervals to ensure that no issue of importance had been omitted (Burnard 1991).

The themes and categories were identified and prioritized through an analysis of their emphasis and intensity (Krueger 1998). The issues the participants considered to be important were repeated at different times throughout the text. These issues were raised either by one individual supported by the other members or by other members re-introducing the topic at different times. The analysis also focused upon whether the comments were spontaneous or if they were in response to a question asked by the researcher. Those issues, which were raised by the group, were given a higher priority.

Stewart and Shamdasani (1990), Burnard (1991), and Morse and Field (1996) all advocate the colour coding of categories. Initially, I attempted to do this, but I found that I had great difficulty with this process. I found it time-consuming, inefficient and, most importantly, with regard to trustworthiness, I found that it isolated comments from the main text. Thus, I abandoned this process and moved on to the next stage, which involved the cutting out and pasting of parts of the text under the different category headings (Burnard 1991) (see Appendix 5 at the end of this chapter). Again, I felt that this fragmented the text and interrupted the flow of the conversation, and I was concerned that the context of the discussion had been altered through the editing process.

My response was to reread and recode the text. I was aware of the risk of the 'precision paradox' (Burnard 1998), whereby researchers, intent upon finding the true nature of the study, overanalyse and so distance themselves from the reality. However, by coding, writing the relevant statements under the appropriate category headings and cross-referencing, I became immersed in the data (Morse and Field 1996) and was able to report the findings in a more meaningful and accurate manner.

## Presenting the findings of the focus group

Writing the findings can be very time-consuming and difficult. You have been immersed in the research for many months and now you are at the stage of trying to crystallize the essence of your findings into a readable, credible report, and this can be a challenge. There are several issues that affect the way you write the report. You need to consider the reader and the reason for the research. If you have conducted this research for submission as part of an educational course, the style of writing required is different from that needed for the publication of an article. However, irrespective of the reader, the presentation must be organized, logical and pull together the emerging themes of the research in a coherent way to give a clear appreciation of the subject.

From the outset of the study, I maintained a diary. I did this to record my difficulties, setbacks and achievements for future reference. It also gave me a record of my feelings and the factors that influenced my progress, which subsequently has formed the basis of this chapter. It was also useful, when I came to analyse the data, because I could consider any events that might have influenced my interpretation. This is important because, unlike quantitative research, you are not relying upon graphs, tables, probability scores etc. to explain the findings. You are attempting to show how you made sense of the descriptive data through a reasonable, fair and trustworthy approach. Ultimately, you are aiming to show how the process you undertook and the results you achieved answered your research question.

Many qualitative researchers write a report using a combination of direct quotations followed by a discussion of the issues raised. Anecdotal evidence is attractive to the reader: it breaks the text, adds interest, gives a feel for what was said and acts to reinforce the writer's interpretation. The difficulty lies in how many quotations to include – too few and they appear sporadic and unconvincing, too many and the reader is left feeling that they are the one doing the interpretation. Furthermore, when using direct quotations, there is always the risk that a participant or clinical area can be identified; therefore, this calls for rigorous attention to detail. This emphasizes the need for the researcher to fully inform the participants before the focus group starts of how the data will be used.

## Conclusion

I hoped to show that my focus groups had in some way enhanced the body of knowledge regarding supervision in practice. I had learned a lot about qualitative research, focus groups and supervision in practice. However, when I compared it to the existing literature, I found that much of my work only reconfirmed what had previously been written. This was somewhat disappointing. On the other hand, what it did allow me to do was consider how I could apply these findings to practice and improve the supervision for the student group that I managed. It also gave me the confidence to make these changes based on the evidence, as opposed to hunches, which is so important in health care.

# Appendix 1

**A study of supervised practice for registered nurses from the perspective of the supervisor and supervisee**

*What is the purpose of the study?*

Supervised practice is an important component of the post-registered course. During supervised practice, it is anticipated that the students apply the theory of ophthalmology to their clinical practice. However, there is very little research to show what actually happens. The aim of this small study is to explore the issue of supervised practice from the viewpoint of the supervisor and supervisee. It is anticipated that the findings from this study will enable me to make any relevant amendments to the documentation issued for use by the supervisors. It will also guide me in preparing future supervisors and supervisees.

*What will be involved if we agree to take part in the study?*

The study is concerned with the staff who have either supervised a course member or who have been supervised during the course, each attending one group discussion session. It is anticipated that the group discussion session will last between one and one-and-a-half hours. Participation in this group discussion is voluntary.

*Can I withdraw from the study at any time?*

Yes, you are free to refuse to join the study and you may withdraw at any time or choose not to discuss certain issues.

*When and where will the interviews take place?*

It is anticipated that the interviews will take place between June and early September.

*What other information will be collected in the study?*

None.

*Will this influence my opportunities to supervise post-registration students in the future?*

No.

*Will the information obtained in this study be confidential?*

Anything you say will be treated in confidence, no names will be mentioned in any reports of the study and care will be taken so that individuals cannot be identified from details in reports of the results of the study.

*Can I complain about the way the study has been conducted?*

If you have any cause to complain about any aspect of the way in which you have been approached or treated during the course of this study, please contact the project co-ordinator, Elaine Stringer. Otherwise you can use the normal university complaints procedure.

# Appendix 2

## Research Consent Form

*Title of Project: A study of supervised practice, for post-registration nurses, from the perspective of the supervisor and supervisee.*

The supervisors/supervisees should each complete the whole of this sheet themselves.

Have you read the Information Sheet?                                    Yes/No

Have you had the opportunity to ask
questions and discuss this study?                                      Yes/No

Have you received a satisfactory answer to your questions?             Yes/No

Have you received enough information about the study?                   Yes/No

Who have you spoken to?

_____

_____

_____

Do you understand that you are free to withdraw from this study

    at any time                                                        Yes/No
    without giving any reason                                          Yes/No
    without affecting your future education                            Yes/No

Do you agree to take part in this study?                               Yes/No

Signed _____

Date: _____

Name in Block Letters _____

# Appendix 3

## Welcome Talk

Hello, and thank you for coming to this focus group session. For the purpose of this session, I am a researcher and, therefore, while I will guide the session, I will not participate in the conversation. My colleague will make notes during the session to ensure the accuracy and objectivity of my reporting. She will not join in the conversation.

The purpose of the session is to gain information about the supervised-practice component of this course. You have experience of being supervised/a supervisor, and we would like to know your point of view, your experience, both positive and negative. There are no right or wrong answers. Please do not worry about what I, my colleague or the other members of the group think. We want to hear from you all: your view is as valuable as anybody else's.

*Please note* that this discussion is being taped. This is for accuracy, objectivity, to ensure that I get all the points noted and to aid analysis. The tapes will only be used for analysis, after which they will be destroyed. Any names on the tape will automatically be deleted to ensure that nobody can be identified. You will be given the opportunity to review the transcripts of this discussion. **You may withdraw from this study now if you do not wish to be taped.**

Please speak up, feel free to give examples or stories to explain a point. Please say what you think. **All data will be treated as confidential.** I have identified four areas for discussion: 'supervision', 'activities', 'preparation' and a category I call 'anything I have missed'. As you discuss these areas, I will be noting down the key points on Post-its, which I will place on the flip charts at the end to summarize the discussion.


Any questions?

# Appendix 4

## Focus Group Guide

Focus Group

Date

Time allocated: 90 minutes

**Welcome**

**Refreshments**

1) Check all participants have read the information sheet and have signed the consent form
2) Read to all the participants (a) the information sheet and (b) the welcome talk information sheet
3) Inform them that their participation is voluntary and they can withdraw at any time. Emphasize the need to maintain confidentiality within the group
4) Test the recording equipment
5) Start the recording and the discussion
6) Summarize the key points and ask the group to confirm or amend
7) Thank all the participants
8) Give information regarding gaining access to the transcripts

# Appendix 5

## Analysis sheet

## Category

| Statement | +ve | -ve | N | Rec | Rpt | Who | I/R | Pg |
|---|---|---|---|---|---|---|---|---|
|  |  |  |  |  |  |  |  |  |

*Key:*
**+ve** – positive statement,
**-ve** – negative statement,
**N** – neutral statement (describing a situation),
**Rec** – a recommendation made by the student,
**Rpt** – was the idea repeated?
**Who** – made this statement?
**I** – intuitive,
**R** – requested by me,
**Pg** – page of the manuscript

# References

Burnard P (1991) A method of analysing interview transcripts in qualitative research. Nurse Education Today 11(7): 461-466.

Burnard P (1998) Challenges in qualitative research in nursing: proceedings of the empowerment and health: an agenda for nurses in the twenty-first century. International Conference held at Brunei, Dasassalam.

Cavanagh S (1998) Content analysis: concepts, methods and applications. Nurse Researcher Compendium 4(2): 178-189.

Greenbaum TL (1998) The Handbook for Focus Group Research. USA: Sage.

Hague PN, Jackson P (1987) Do Your Own Market Research. London: Kogan Page.

Krueger RA (1998) Moderating Focus Groups. Focus Group Kit 4. London: Sage.

Marshall C, Rossman GB (1999) Designing Qualitative Research. London: Sage.

Morgan DL (1997) Focus Group as Qualitative Research (second edition). London: Sage.

Morgan DL (1998a) The Focus Group Guidebook. Focus Group Kit 1. USA: Sage.

Morgan DL (1998b) Planning Focus Groups. Focus Group Kit 2. USA: Sage.

Morgan DL, Krueger RA (1993) When to use focus groups and why. In Morgan DL (ed.) Successful Focus Groups: advancing the state of the art. Newbury Park, Ca.: Sage.

Morse JM (1989) Qualitative Nursing Research: a contemporary dialogue. Chicago, Ill: Aspen Publishers.

Morse JM, Field PA (1996) Nursing Research: the application of qualitative approaches. Royston, Herts.: Chapman Hall.

Polit DF, Hungler BP (1997) Essentials of Nursing Research, Methods, Appraisal and Utilisation (third edition). Philadelphia, Pa: Lippincott.

Proctor S (1998) Linking philosophy and method in the nursing process: the case for realism. Nurse Researcher 5(4): 121-126.

Sloan G (1998) Focus group interviews: defining clinical supervision. Nursing Standard 12(42): 40-43.

Stewart DW, Shamdasani PN (1990) Focus Groups: theory and practice. London: Sage.

# CHAPTER THREE

# Action research

LOUISE RIGG

## Introduction

The difficulty in teaching health professionals the basic principles of good infection-control practice, the lack of knowledge about infection control and the ongoing problem of health professionals' non-compliance with basic hygiene in hospitals cause grave concern. Individual clinicians, who may be aware of potential infection-control problems in their speciality, have no reliable means to judge their own practice against standard rates or acceptable thresholds for hospital-acquired infection. Some hospital-acquired infection is unavoidable, owing to patient and environmental risk factors, but there is evidence of effective hospital-infection-control programmes with reductions of hospital-acquired infections being reported of around 30%. Despite advances in medicine, technology, treatment techniques, control of infection methods and a scientific understanding of the aetiology and epidemiology of infection, control of hospital-acquired infection continues to cause concern. To date, there are no comparative data about the effectiveness of infection control in the UK. The full extent of the impact of hospital-acquired infection on a patient's short- and long-term experiences is not measured in the UK. The problem of hospital infection is recognized by all involved in health care today. All the evidence suggests that effective infection control would improve quality of care, reduce costs and prevent deaths in the NHS.

Evidence exists for the effective prevention of hospital-acquired infection, yet this evidence is not being applied in practice. The barriers to delivering effective hospital infection control are increasing: technology is expanding, risks to patients are greater and resources are constrained. This chapter recounts the experiences of a clinical researcher who was determined to explore the real world of infection control in nursing practice. This research explored a novel, practical and resource-effective approach to applying empirical evidence in practice by developing and evaluating a comprehensive prospective method for a bedside audit of hospital-acquired infection in patients requiring intensive care. The research sought to stimulate and develop nursing practice of effective infection control with particular emphasis being placed on the role of nurses. In essence, the research tested the potential for nurses to adopt a central co-ordinating role for infection control within nursing care.

While the methodology to determine the impact of the interventions on patient outcome was quantitative in nature – based upon robust epidemiological principles – the research focused on behavioural change and was underpinned by the exploratory use of action research and the application of Lewin's Theory of Change. This meant that, while no precise outcome was expected or guaranteed, the researcher set out with a specific purpose, that of developing, implementing and testing a method for a bedside audit of infection acquired by patients requiring intensive care. The research was initiated as a methodological evaluative pragmatic study that adopted a time series intervention drawing on both quantitative and qualitative research methodologies. The focus was on monitoring outcomes rather than explaining factors that may or may not have been changed by the interventions: information gathering, responsive education and an audit of infection with a feedback of results.

## Action research

Action research provides a clinically focused approach to change management utilizing Lewin's Theory of Change. This method closely matched the researcher's personal philosophy about the change process. The emphasis was to be on professional and practice development. The end product for effective infection-control programmes must always be the behavioural components of practice, for instance improved hand hygiene and evidence-based care of invasive therapies and devices. Therefore, use of action research using a naturalistic, intuitive approach was considered a valid approach to a clinical problem that requires practice development through use of psychosocial influencing tactics provided within an educational framework. The emphasis in this study was on testing theory derived from evidence of large-scale research conducted outside the UK and exploring the potential for improvements in quality of care and impact on patient outcome in the ICU before recommending future strategies for infection control. Local objectives were to promote the ownership and control of audit information, improve documentation of clinical information related to acquired infection, improve the clinical information base, support the identification of local infection-control problems, inform and educate staff, aid decision-making and influence changes in clinical practice.

The total research programme spans over ten years. Originally, the researcher began to study the problem of infection within a large general intensive care unit (Inglis et al. 1992a, 1992b, 1993). Although the proportion of patients requiring intensive care is small, these patients account for the largest proportion of hospital-acquired infection, have the highest morbidity and mortality, and represent the highest cost to the health service. A national survey of infection-control policies and practices in intensive care units (ICUs) in the UK was undertaken (Inglis et al. 1992a) and a modular infection-control education programme was developed, incorporating a systematic approach to preventing ICU-acquired infection (Sproat and Inglis 1992). A number of infection-control-practice developments in the ICU were facilitated, but initiatives did not include routine audit of patient outcome for infection.

## Research parameters

Within the Trust where this research was being undertaken, there was an increased awareness of the quality and cost implications of hospital-acquired infections. The researcher was asked to present a paper that analysed the infection-control services in the Trust. This was developed into a successful research proposal submitted to Yorkshire Region Research and Development Directorate that allowed the research to be extended for a full two years and built upon previous knowledge and experience gained through working on the intensive care unit. The objective of the study was to determine the benefits of targeted surveillance of a group of high-risk general surgical patients, using routine clinical data with feedback of results going to nursing and managerial staff. The programme was complemented by using structured questionnaires to research issues relating nursing education, nurses' knowledge and practice of infection control and their attitudes towards infection control in the Trust. As a result of the infection audit and the questionnaire responses, a research-based modular education programme was introduced for clinical nurses in two of four surgical wards.
　　Research interventions included an audit of the four site-specific infections, pilot ward questionnaire distribution and analysis, feedback of results to staff on pilot wards, feedback of results to managers and the introduction of an infection-control educational programme on the pilot wards. The researcher also worked as a staff nurse on the two pilot wards during the first post-intervention period. Primary data, obtained from the computerized patient administration system (PAS), identified all discharged patients from the four general surgical wards during the three data collection periods. This included collection of demographic data, risk factors, significant health care interventions and any documented

indications of clinical infection. Clinical indicators for each site-specific infection were recorded in four parameters (clinical signs and symptoms of infection, positive bacteriology culture result, new or changed antibiotic prescription and written medical diagnosis of infection) and were combined to determine patient outcome. Infections occurring more than 48 hours after admission were defined as hospital-acquired.

Results were aggregated for each three-month data collection period, providing baseline pre-intervention measurements of hospital-acquired infection and two subsequent post-intervention measurements for comparison purposes. Infection rates were calculated for the study group of high-risk surgical patients discharged from the four surgical wards and expressed as a percentage of patients affected by one or more hospital-acquired infections, the overall percentage of all four hospital-acquired infections and the incidence of each site-specific hospital-acquired infection. Average percentage reduction in the incidence of all four site-specific hospital-acquired infections from baseline to the second post-intervention measurement across the four wards was 59% (from 30.58% to 12.64%) and from baseline to the first post-intervention measurement was 49% (from 30.58% to 15.69%).

## Pilot and control wards

An interesting pattern of results occurred in two of the wards. One was a pilot ward and one a control ward. These two wards remained more closely matched than the other two. During the first post-intervention period, nurses on the control ward conducted their own ward-based audit of surgical-wound infection on behalf of the team of surgeons. This audit occurred outside the research study and lasted for one month and was then discontinued. During the first post-intervention period, nurses on the control ward conducted their own ward-based audit of surgical-wound infection on behalf of the team of surgeons. Results indicate that the ward-based audit of surgical-wound infection on the control ward had an immediate impact on reducing rates of all four hospital-acquired infections in that ward. Findings suggest that the internally managed ward-based data collection on the control ward had a stronger impact on patient outcome of infection, in the short term, as opposed to external data collection conducted by the nurse researcher on the pilot ward. The control ward had the greatest reduction in the percentage of infected patients and the incidence of the four site-specific hospital-acquired infections during the first pre-intervention period (when audit activities had taken place).

Questionnaire responses emphasized the difficulties nurses have in integrating infection-control knowledge in their routine clinical practice.

Findings suggested that nurses have a poor knowledge and understanding of how the principles of microbiology or infection control could be applied in practice. The study revealed nurses' lack of awareness of their potential role in infection control and confusion over recommended infection-control policies and procedures. Nurses generally accepted that they needed to improve both knowledge and infection-control practice, but there was a lack of time and resources for study on the wards. Nurses on the pilot wards freely discussed their lack of knowledge and their own and others' variable practices in infection control. Nurses generally wanted more practical information on effective infection control. The results identified specific problems and provided a basis for improvements in infection control.

The method provided a framework for case-mix identification, case definition, data collection and identification of indicators for measurement of hospital-acquired infection. This study was well supported by hospital managers, who responded to the results by incorporating them within a successful business case increasing the infection-control team by employing an additional four senior infection-control nurses. Using a retrospective approach to an audit of hospital-acquired infection revealed a number of problems; yet, despite the difficulties experienced, the research programme was well accepted by the staff.

## Influencing nurses to use valid research

Building on the available research evidence and local experience, it became obvious that nurses could make a greater contribution to effective infection control but that multiple strategies would be required to influence their compliance with infection-control recommendations. Ideal strategies would incorporate an audit of infection with feedback of rates to nursing staff with appropriate, responsive infection-control education. Sustained change would require the transfer of the problems, issues and potential solutions to nurses. The focus would need to be on the nurse's role and nursing infection-control clinical practices. The knowledge and skills gained from the research programme led to the development of a research proposal to develop and test a prospective method of auditing infections acquired by patients requiring intensive care. The confidential nature of infection data collected nationally means that not all clinical staff who are involved in studies are aware of the local results.

The observations made within previous studies and further reviews of the literature influenced the development of the action research programme, which aimed to adopt a practical, clinically useful approach to the problem of hospital-acquired infection and infection control. The researcher wanted to develop a system to routinely audit hospital-acquired infection that supported an increase in knowledge and facilitated infection-control practice development without relying on expert infection control input or major additional resources. The proposed bedside audit of hospital-acquired infections would incorporate modified definitions for hospital-acquired infections and provide the means of prospectively auditing risk factors, process measures and outcome for infection within routine documentation. The research programme aimed to develop an acceptable, reliable method to audit the incidence of four categories of site-specific infection acquired by patients in intensive care units. These infections are lower-respiratory-tract infection (LRTI), blood-stream infection (BSI), surgical-wound infection (SWI) and catheter-related urinary-tract infection (UTI).

In order to achieve this three key goals need to be achieved:

1. identification and agreement of a clinical data set to audit four categories of site-specific ICU-acquired infection
2. development of a protocol for clinical audit of the four ICU-acquired infections, using routinely collected clinical data and to develop this protocol within an effective audit tool
3. evaluation of the staff response to the audit

The system of audit developed for this research was applied to all patients admitted to two research sites from two different health regions, involving a total study population of over 2,000 patients. General approval for the study was gained from ICU nurses and doctors, the infection control team (ICT) and members of relevant hospital management teams. Arranging formal clinical access and ethical approval involved gaining access and permission to use hospital data, clinical ICU data and microbiology data in both paper-based and computerized format. Approval was given for plans for data protection, data security and data-management plans, including the proposed data analysis, presentation and research dissemination. Feedback of infection incidence was continuous during the period of research. Incidence of hospital-acquired infections was measured using nurses to collect and co-ordinate data collection. All research interventions and infection-control educational activities introduced within this study were supported and facilitated by the researcher. Data collection for each patient included risk assessment with the collation of routine clinical and microbiological data and objective measurement of patient outcome combining clinical and microbiological data variables. The research sought to test the integration of the data items into a practical audit tool for measuring the incidence of hospital-acquired infection in a rigorous, scientific way and was directed at implementing evidence-based infection-control practice. The research study sought to answer the research questions posed before design of the study. Data analysis aimed to describe and summarize the results and test the hypothesis that the audit would affect behaviour, resulting in reduced infection rates.

## The two research areas

This section describes the activities in the two ICUs that adopted and tested the full infection-control care planning and audit system. The pilot site was a six-bed paediatric intensive care unit (PICU), and the other site was an eight-bed general adult intensive therapy unit (GITU). The researcher collated additional background information that explored the available ICU information sources that might be used for the research data collection. Before any research interventions or educational sessions, a questionnaire was distributed to all ICU staff. It used semi-structured questions to investigate nurses' infection-control education and knowledge and their attitudes towards infection control and microbiology. It questioned staff on their use of infection control within patient assessment and care planning. It also allowed staff to give their suggestions for improving infection control in three key areas: infection control in their ICU, communication of infection-control policies and infection-control education, and allowed suggestions for topics to be incorporated within an education programme for the ICU.

All research interventions and infection-control educational activities introduced within this study were introduced, supported and facilitated by the researcher. During the research, sufficient time was allowed for a group of nurses to volunteer to support this research programme. After a period of educational and audit training seminars, nurses were asked to collect data on the incidence of four site-specific ICU-acquired infections, utilizing secondary sources of routinely collected clinical and microbiological data recorded in the computerized clinical and pathology information systems and within patients' case notes.

This complete system for infection-control care planning and audit did not require special expertise or knowledge for determining patient outcome for ICU-acquired infection. For both ICUs, there was an introductory period involving communication with staff agreeing the infection-control care plans that were modified to local specifications. Data were collected by nursing staff at the bedside, while clinical and microbiological data from primary ICU sources, that is from nursing and medical records and associated computerized clinical information systems for each patient admitted to the unit, were also used. Prospective data collection used ICU nursing staff to manage data collection, collation and communication within the ICU. Significant intensive care interventions and patient outcome events were documented and variations in these processes identified. The complete coded audit and care planning system included the following stages:

- patient risk assessment for ICU-acquired infection
- following or adapting a standard ICU-specific infection-control care plan
- daily evaluation of patient infection status
- recording positive outcome indicators for each infection in four parameters
- recording patient outcome for each of the four ICU-acquired infections

# Defining an ICU-acquired infection

An ICU-acquired infection was identified as an infection that was not present or incubating at the time of admission. ICU-acquired infections occur 48 to 72 hours after admission to the ICU.

# Staging site-specific infection

Development of an ICU-acquired infection needed to be made explicit within the documentation and during data collection. Generally, the stages followed the infection processes that nurses would, or should, readily know. The research documentation included guidance for staff on the associated clinical signs and symptoms that may occur for each site-specific ICU-acquired infection.

| Stage | General infection status |
|---|---|
| 0 | Patient at risk – no positive indication of infection |
| 1 | Possible pre-infectious indicators of infection |
| 2 | Probable indications of infection |
| 3 | Actual infection |

# Objective measurement of patient outcome

For each site-specific infection being measured, coding combined the stages of infection with four parameters. The parameters to be measured were:

1. clinical signs and symptoms of infection
2. positive bacteriology results
3. change of antibiotic
4. written medical diagnosis of infection

# Experiences from the PICU

## Theoretical framework for change

The PICU nurse manager decided that one senior nurse would have the role of PICU research co-ordinator, internally managing the project as part of her individual performance review. The PICU research co-ordinator was visited frequently, and a satisfactory initial working relationship was established. It is reasonable to say the PICU research co-ordinator was a reluctant 'volunteer'. Both researcher and the PICU research co-ordinator agreed to continue with the project. The role of the researcher was to facilitate the PICU research co-ordinator in familiarizing herself with the research literature, and a resource file was provided by the researcher that covered relevant infection-control literature with specific emphasis on the prevention of infection in the ICU. A series of PICU nursing staff seminars contributed to the change process by incorporating the background to the research (the problem) and the results of previous research (identifying potential for change) with education and awareness-raising information (providing the means for change). The research problem was presented within the context of the PICU, and the need for change was discussed. Desired changes were suggested and negotiated with staff. The seminars gave staff who attended feedback on the results of the staff questionnaires on infection-control education, knowledge and practice. Release of nursing staff from the PICU was problematic, so the research seminars were given in the central area of the PICU during a normal shift. A period of careful planning and negotiation continued to take place through regular meetings, and the research co-ordinator established an internal team of nurse associates who became the PICU infection-control quality-improvement team. Independent of the researcher, but assisted by the infection-control research resources, this internal team established priorities for the PICU. The PICU initially developed an information booklet for parents on infection control on the PICU and proceeded to develop an educational programme for staff.

## Disseminating the documentation

The next stage of the research process was to disseminate the proposed research documentation and to develop a PICU-specific infection-control core care plan. The documentation was designed and developed to support the collection and collation of infection-control risk factors for four ICU-acquired infections. The PICU research co-ordinator organized all nursing and medical staff to review this documentation, and modifications were made accordingly. Achieving consensus for the PICU research documentation and the PICU infection-control care plan required an intense period of consultation with members of the PICU team and health professionals working outside the PICU who had responsibility for infection control.

## Developing consensus

Consensus was achieved for the research documentation, which included the PICU infection-control care plan and the PICU infection control risk-assessment tool. The PICU infection control summary chart was incorporated after requests from medical staff made during the pilot phase. Research documentation was supported by an introduction to the research, which was written to promote staff and parental understanding of the research. A referenced background to the research was presented as an appendix to the PICU research documentation.

## Developing the documentation

Nursing, medical and microbiology staff agreed the infection definitions and research documentation. The PICU research documentation was developed to support daily monitoring of each child's infection status, relevant interventions and outcome. Infections measured were LRTIs, BSIs, SWIs and UTIs. A clinical outcome summary sheet was provided for all four site-specific infections being measured. Definitions for all four site-specific infections were adapted from previously published, nationally acceptable definitions that had been used for previous research studies. All research interventions and infection-control educational activities introduced within this study were supported and facilitated by the researcher.

## Managing bedside data collection

Each folder had the contact name, address and telephone number of the researcher, research supervisors and external advisors to the action research. One box file contained new research documentation and one box file was used to store completed research documentation. The research co-ordinator took full responsibility for managing documentation collection and collation. Staff were asked to implement the following procedures for all children admitted to the PICU:

1. complete infection risk assessment on admission
2. complete processes
3. stages outcomes documentation once daily at midnight
4. complete a discharge summary at the end of a child's PICU stay

**Piloting the bedside infection-control care planning and audit**

The researcher visited the PICU frequently but in reality was not required to manage the research. The methodology for data collection was not changed, but the research documentation was modified slightly as a result of evaluation by nursing staff.

**Research development**

With the encouragement of the PICU's medical director, the research co-ordinator prepared and presented interim results of the research at an international medical conference. When the planned research period was complete, the system was adapted in response to previous results and the increasing demands on PICU nursing staff. In 1998, the research co-ordinator was successful in gaining the position of research nurse, managing and co-ordinating a national UK drugs trial relating to meningococcal infection. The PICU-acquired infection study is now completely owned and managed by the PICU. The researcher's previous experiences suggested that data collection by nurses at the bedside, in collaboration with medical staff, proved successful. Therefore, increased potential for change might be achieved when action research, practice development and change management were combined using a quantitative approach to using clinical information to audit infections.

# Experiences from the GITU

Initial access to the GITU was obtained by inviting the infection control doctor and the infection control nurse from the Trust to a University of Sheffield post-graduate seminar given by the researcher in September 1995. At this point, the ICT agreed to give their support to the action research programme. The introductory stage of the research in the GITU lasted six months, from December 1995 to May 1996. Initial contact with the GITU was through the senior nurse manager, who arranged for a small group of senior sisters to attend a research seminar and to consider whether to proceed with the research programme in the GITU. After this seminar, it was decided to present the research to the rest of the senior team for a collective decision to be made about progressing with the research in their unit. While the researcher thought that full agreement and clinical access had been arranged with all members of the clinical management team, one consultant was overlooked. This posed problems later in the study when authorization for access to medical records required this individual's permission. This problem was quickly resolved by writing to the consultant in question and making a follow-up telephone call. This resulted in full permission for access being given. Ethical approval was given as a result of a full submission to the Ethical Committee of the Trust.

## Theoretical framework for change

The management of the research programme in the GITU was different from that in the PICU, but the researcher continued to use the theoretical framework of action research and Lewin's Theory of Change adapted to facilitate changes in the PICU. In contrast to the PICU, the researcher had no previous contact with the GITU, but there was a strong management team with proactive support and encouragement of staff development, education and practice developments.

## Unfreezing: coming to terms with the need for change

There was a system for routine bacteriology sampling of patients three times per week, and there was an infection control link nurse established on the GITU. This nurse had already undertaken an infection-control course, and it was usual for nurses to be sent on this course as part of their professional development. Although the infection control link nurses left the GITU during this study, there was a replacement infection control link nurse, ensuring continuity throughout the research programme. In addition, a charge nurse from GITU had been seconded to the ICT and there was a positive attitude to infection control from most members of the GITU team. It was accepted that the ICT was overworked and that an additional resource in the GITU was welcomed. As a result of information gathering on the GITU, the researcher decided, primarily because of the differing nature of work in the GITU from that in the PICU, that rather than having a GITU research co-ordinator who was responsible for the research the researcher would maintain a high profile in the GITU. The researcher was well supported by the infection control link nurse, the senior sisters, nursing team and the nurse manager on the GITU. The ICT and staff from the pathology department were encouraging towards the research and were willing to review the research protocol and provide the computerized pathology data. Five introductory research seminars were presented from January 1996 to March 1996 giving background to the research and presenting the results of the questionnaires.

## Introducing new values

The GITU was a much larger unit than the PICU. Early discussions about the potential of the action research programme being introduced in the

GITU included demonstrating the PICU research documentation. Despite the positive attitude of GITU nurses to infection control and an apparent recognition of its importance to nursing practice, there was concern from senior nurses about GITU nurses at the bedside having to complete more paperwork. Nurses already recorded bacteriology results on a single communication sheet in the patient's case notes, but there was no information about infection rates in the GITU. This one factor, the opportunity to measure GITU-acquired infection, seemed to be the convincing element to developing acceptance of the research programme. Nurses were to give their time to test and evaluate the research documentation. The research was promoted as an opportunity to explore whether the research evidence, derived from outside the UK, could be implemented and shown to be effective in this country. Again, with many nurses involved in their own further education, there were many opportunities to promote the action research programme as an educational opportunity for nurses, regardless of the final outcome.

### Acceptance of new values

An internal ICT was set up to support the research and to aid research communication. The researcher maintained responsibility for the administration of the research and was given valuable assistance by the GITU team in organizing the educational seminars, in encouraging staff to attend seminars and in actively promoting the completion of the bedside research documentation. An important difference in the GITU compared with the PICU was that the series of educational seminars gave the researcher greater exposure to larger numbers of GITU staff. The seminars also ensured that all nurses were made aware not only of the research programme but also of the role and responsibility of nurses in preventing infection.

### Developing consensus

Because of the concerns expressed about GITU workloads and the potential additional paperwork involved in the PICU-style research documentation, the development of the documentation differed from that on the PICU. In the GITU it was acknowledged that nurses would not be motivated to go through a series of documentation, so a modified version was redesigned and developed within a limited number of pages. This contained all the essential stages and elements recognized in the research protocol. Again, an intense period of work was needed by the researcher to develop a GITU-specific infection-control care plan and infection control risk-assessment tool. The documentation was supported by written research information, and documentation was developed to support the collection and collation of infection risk factors, process measures of care on a summary chart and clinical outcome for four GITU-acquired infections. An infection control communication sheet was provided for additional comments by nursing staff. A copy of the documentation was displayed on the staff notice board and everyone was asked to consider this and make comments. Consensus for the system was achieved, which included the infection control doctor reviewing the full documentation and agreeing to its use in practice. There was general consensus that the data covered all items required for effective infection control.

### Developing the documentation

Infections measured in GITU were LRTIs, BSIs, UTIs and SWIs.

### Managing bedside data collection

A system was agreed for GITU data collection and collation of results and followed the steps taken in the PICU (see above).

### Piloting the bedside infection-control care planning and audit

Bedside collection of data commenced in June 1996. The methodology for data collection was not changed from original plans, but the research documentation was modified slightly as a result of pilot evaluation by nursing staff. Changes were made to the risk-assessment process chart, and the communication page was added after the pilot.

### Establishing staff satisfaction and ownership

The general response to the audit was positive; staff made comments such as 'we feel involved' and that the researcher was 'not just a voice on the end of the telephone'. There was some resistance to increasing the amount of documentation, which was difficult to quantify, but the researcher endeavoured to be available to nurses who were having difficulty in completing the forms. Completion of the audit documentation revealed a problem with communication in the GITU: nurses did not know the results of cultures until they were filing the paper records, but a microbiologist visited the GITU every morning to report the results verbally. Nurses realized they were being missed from this aspect of communication. They were not normally included in this process, which was usually between the medical microbiologist and the GITU doctor. Some nurses acted to make sure they were included in the feedback of results, but this remained problematic.

The researcher asked for the daily print-outs from the microbiology laboratory to be left and filed on the GITU, but this did not become routine practice.

## Evaluation of the education programme

Each of nine educational infection control seminars were presented twice. A Likert scale was used to evaluate the impact of each session. Each member of staff attending was asked to identify if they agreed or disagreed with statements that evaluated the seminar. A total of 80 staff attended the nine seminars, and 63 evaluations were completed for eight of the nine sessions.

## Evaluation of the bedside audit

In October 1996, after three months of a bedside audit, 18 staff returned interim audit evaluation questionnaires and 17 listed both positive and negative points about the documentation for infection-control care planning and audit. One nurse did not list any positive points. Seventeen nurses wanted to continue the audit as a research project, 15 thought there was sufficient time to complete the documentation, six wanted more information or help to assist in completing the forms, but 11 did not. Nine staff wanted to keep the system as it was, without changes, five did not. Nine would keep the current system but change it in some way. Thirteen nurses felt that the infection control audit should become a permanent part of the patient's record.

## GITU research development

Data feedback was given to staff at an interim stage and at a series of seminars to present and discuss final results. Graphs, charts and explanatory comments were displayed on the notice board in the coffee room. As in a previous study, nurses did not at first grasp the graphical representations and welcomed the interpretation of the results. One health care assistant announced that, after seeing the graphical displays, she did not want to join the results seminar as she would not be able to understand but after being coaxed into the seminar was pleased to announce that she did now understand. A project team was created to determine how best to use the results of the research. A team was set up to look at documentation, education and audit. Because there were no major changes in infection rates as a result of the bedside audit, it was agreed not to pursue this route but to develop a care planning document for all patients that would form part of their routine documentation for care planning, communication and with a prompt sheet for risk factors and definitions for acquired infection.

The GITU also used a computerized care planning system, and a problem and evaluation sheet was written into this system for routine use in daily care planning. Infection control planning and evaluation started at completion of the study (June 1997). Bacteriology data were analysed in date order, for individual patients and by bacteria cultured. Both paper and electronic versions of the data were provided. It was thought that it would be useful to include these data with the main GITU database and include patterns of antibiotic usage with patterns of antibiotic resistance.

### GITU research dissemination

The researcher presented results of the research at a multidisciplinary study day organized by the GITU. This included presentations by the GITU medical consultants, the researcher and two GITU sisters who presented results of qualitative studies in the GITU.

### Future research and development plans

The discussion at the study day became a catalyst for a collaborative research project undertaken for the clinical management team (CMT) within the GITU. This programme of research focused on two aspects of critical care; one was to explore the potential for nurses to discharge patients from the HDU and the other was an audit of at-risk patients in the general wards. Both projects were led by nurses on behalf of the CMT and were facilitated by the researcher during 1998 and 1999. From 1997, research results have been disseminated by the researcher at five national nursing conferences, two regional conferences and two further conferences in 1999, one being a symposium.

# Conclusion

The most efficient infection surveillance methods developed for the UK are too time-consuming for practical use. This means there is no convincing evidence on which to support recommendations for change in education, clinical practice or research. Reduction of hospital-acquired infection relies on improvements in infection control – such as handwashing or improved care of invasive medical devices – but health professionals have difficulty learning and integrating this knowledge in practice. Clinical practice of infection control, particularly handwashing, is sub-optimal, and health professionals appear to be resistant to changing their infection-control practice. The problem of hospital infection and the difficulties in its effective control are well recognized, and research-based recommendations have been made for changing clinical practice. Infection surveillance combined with responsive infection control methods have been shown to be the most effective way to reduce rates of infection. However, implementation of these changes is proving difficult to achieve in the UK. Workloads in the NHS are rising, resources are limited, there is a lack of useful clinical information and limited use of information technology to provide knowledge-based systems that can guide practice, education and management for infection control.

McCormack (1999a) discusses a model for implementing research into practice, describes factors for success and proposes that service improvement is a function of the strength of the evidence base, the context or prevailing culture and appropriate facilitation. He describes the factors within an interactive, dynamic matrix that can be used to identify and analyse practice development projects. Using McCormack's framework for analysis, the strength of the evidence in this study was high, but not of the highest order of randomized controlled trials.

The context and prevailing culture of each ICU was clear. It was patient-focused and multidisciplinary with prevailing medical dominance. The educational culture had a strong image of professionalism. In presenting the evidence to clinical staff, success was achieved in agreement with McCormack's (1999b) 'enabling factors' for practice development. The researcher was sensitive to and aware of the specialist nature of intensive care nursing, and saw the evident need for nursing involvement in the project. There was a growing awareness to both clinical- and cost-effectiveness issues and a commitment to individual- and team-nursing development. The overall aim was one of practitioner ownership with management support. Changes were approached systematically and were in support of an established professional vision of practice development and evidence-based nursing practice. There were political overtones to the facilitation of the changes with promotion of the role of ICU nurses as highly specialized, intelligent and unique. The issue of ICU nurses' potential replacement by technical staff and NVQ-level trained assistants was recognized by ICU staff. With this in mind, involvement in the research was promoted as a means of demonstrating the implicit actions of qualified nurses. Nursing actions emphasized were risk assessment, risk management and those aimed at the prevention of infection. This highlighted the case for retaining highly skilled qualified nurses within the ICU.

Continuing in the use of McCormack's model for identifying successful implementation of research into practice (McCormack 1999b), development achieved in this study was predominantly an attitudinal change to ICU-acquired infection, ICU infection control and the role of ICU nurses in infection control. There was evidence of an increasing confidence in the nurses' competence and understanding, with nurses gaining a deeper understanding of the significance of bacteriology results for care. There was a clear focus on nursing care processes with development of clinical leadership in practice development. In common with Hope (1998), the researcher had been active in practice development long before her awareness of the appropriateness of the theoretical framework of action research.

Again in common with Hope (1998), the researcher had been initially frustrated with being unable to proceed with a particular form of research (the controlled trial) and gained 'energy' from the paradigm of action research, which Hope describes as 'characterised by decisions trails and logistics which are context bound, complex and open to confusion'. In considering this description, he expresses concern that the existing literature on action research generally understates its complexity. He argues that actions are not 'neat and linear', which generates a problem when trying to describe the process of action research using an accepted academic approach. He uses the analogy of action research as a journey involving change, and which is a 'serendipitous' process involving areas of language and discourse, activities and practices and social relationships and organization. Hope (1998) cites Waterman (1994), who argues that the problems of defining action research can be seen as a symbol for 'artistry and flexibility in the practice of nursing and action research'. In analysing the facilitation skills used in this research, the action taken took similar but slightly different approaches in each ICU. The role was one of external facilitator to an internal ICU facilitator which sought to be flexible and collaborative, while at times needing to be directive and persuasive. Strong emphasis was placed on the importance and relevance of the educative and developmental processes for nurses and nursing.

# Researcher's experiences

The researcher's experiences in this study were in agreement with Titchen (1999), who, in discussing her role as external facilitator in a long-term action research project, describes her relationship with clinical staff as one of a 'critical companion', being sensitive to needs and responsive to differing individuals and groups. Using the accepted theoretical framework of critical social science, she described practice development as a process of integrating 'professional nursing craft knowledge' with a research base. Titchen describes the relationship between a practice development facilitator and that of a nurse being facilitated; this requires respect, mutuality, reciprocity with demonstration of 'living out shared values and beliefs' within a process of 'learning from practice'. While facilitation in this study took both directive and flexible approaches, there were elements of the four components that were highly influential in the personal qualities of an individual change agent: personal, interpersonal, intellectual and educational. In this study, all these qualities were utilized and the relationships built with the internal ICU change agents were and are sustained on both personal and professional levels. Hope (1998) holds the opinion that most nurses are equipped with the skills necessary for action research: 'having well developed interpersonal skills, flexibility to respond to new situations, a degree of social entrepreneurialism, a willingness to listen to alternative views and the ability to be reflective and reflexive'.

## Action research: some conclusions

Action research provided a flexible approach that suited the adaptation of the researcher's views on infection control in intensive care units and translated what is regarded as an academic and scientific subject into practical clinical terms. Put another way, knowledge gained about the prevention and management of infection within this research was derived from clinical practice with changes occurring at the interface of patients and their carers.

Action research was used to determine the potential for change, to introduce change and to understand the nature of that change. It used an intuitive approach favoured by nurses, who see the value of education, practice development and who generally focus on the nursing processes of care. Nurses find difficulty in defining outcomes of care and identifying or demonstrating the relationships between processes of care and patient outcomes. This was borne out by the results of the GITU audit evaluation when nurses were asked about potential positive benefits of the audit. Most comments related to improving care and raising awareness of infection and infection control. Few nurses responded that knowing rates of infection was a positive benefit to them. The highest anxiety that nurses felt when considering involvement in the research and evaluating its impact was the time taken for completion of the audit, problems of missing data items and concerns over having to complete more paperwork. Using action research and Lewin's Theory of Change enabled the researcher to validate previous approaches to change interventions and support her personal view as sustainable change being part of a slow incremental process. The research was promoted as an act of faith without any preconceived end points. Being open with staff and promoting the use of action research, or real clinical research, contained an educational element for the staff. It introduced a partnership, or bond, between researcher and motivated staff. Action research was seen as a process rather than a means to an end and certainly gave focus to the research and drew considerable attention to the processes involved. In both ICUs, there was an emphasis on infection-control education and its intrinsic value. Even if the research proved inconclusive, there would be a benefit in that nurses would have clinical information about local problems that could be used to promote practice development.

Many nurses were involved in education programmes and the research was able to bring alive some of the theories introduced in the classroom. The researcher had considerable experience in this field of study but was conscious that imposed change without negotiation is not welcome by current NHS staff. Within this study, in contrast to many new projects introduced into the NHS, at all points of this research, ICU staff were given control. While senior nurses actively promoted data collection, the approach was to promote the involvement in the research as voluntary. There was little change in plans, but ample opportunity was offered to all grades and groups of staff to allow changes to be made. Conducting research in the NHS has many challenges, and researchers need powers of persuasion while at the same time they have to uphold the rights of patients and clinical staff. At any stage, one member of the wider team in a hospital could withhold consent to proceed. In contrast to the open, unstructured approach to change taken using the action research, the fact that the researcher had personal funding for the doctoral study from the Nursing Directorate of the Department of Health meant that the research process needed to be structured. Fortunately, the research problem lent itself well to a structured approach to evaluative research. The research design followed a classic approach in its development. There was problem identification and the development of a research question, with aims, objectives and hypothesis with statistical considerations being made. This was a considerable asset when seeking and gaining support from the medical clinicians, the ICT and particularly when applying for ethical approval for the study. The predominant concern of the medical team on the PICU was the use of non-published, non-validated definitions. But they were persuaded that the research was exploratory in nature and that gold-standards do not exist in the UK for defining hospital-acquired infection. It was emphasized that the focus of the research was on the clinical utility of the audit balanced by clinical validity and reliability. The immediate need was to address clinical problems, to develop user-friendly methods of data collection and to develop further research programmes to test and validate the methods. Full analysis of the data was not completed but will eventually be used within the development of the research programme. Immediate action will be to disseminate the research methods and results. The general lessons learnt from this innovation in practice will be considered. Further research is planned to test the approach in other units and to determine the cost and potential benefits. Research data are computerized and maintained in such a way that further validation of the accuracy of the measurement can be made. The contribution of risk factors to the development of infection will be explored. Data will be analysed to provide an audit trail of events that will indicate the time from first signs and symptoms of infection (and possibly pre-infectious indicators) to the first sample taking, first bacteriology result and first therapeutic intervention.

Measurement of ICU-acquired infection provided useful information for future local comparison purposes, and the data showed trends of infection over time, identifying problems in each ICU, and provided a basis for quality improvement initiatives in ICUs. The documentation was designed to collect and collate only routine items of clinical information that the nurse at the bedside on an ICU would already know or be able to gather in a very short time. The actual recording of data should in reality pose a negligible burden on nurses who are constantly by the bedside in the ICU. While the results do not indicate general improvement in patient outcome occurring over time, the method of data collection was applied systematically and rigorously. Regardless of the difficulties in applying the protocol and controlling the study, measurement of hospital-acquired infection rates provided useful information for future local comparison purposes. However, the reliability and validity of the results should be weighed against their potential clinical utility. Accepting the limitations of this study, the approach taken has potential application for surveillance of endemic hospital-acquired infections in a wide range of clinical specialities. The system provided a framework for case-mix identification, case definitions, data collection and the identification of indicators for the measurement of ICU-acquired infection that can be adapted to meet specific requirements of different clinical situations and which is directly related to improving patient outcome. It was shown to be feasible to incorporate the audit tool within routine documentation of clinical care in a systematic way and with apparent cost-efficiency. Cost-effectiveness was not formally tested. There was, of course, input from the researcher who was supported full-time on a studentship and provided time and resources to initiate the study, develop documentation and educational resources. There was also, for the purpose of the research, ICU staff time needed for development and management. No additional test or interventions were required; the impact was the adherence to routine systematic risk assessment, with more responsive care planning, which should have contributed to improving the prevention and management of infection control in the ICU.

# The practical applications of successful action research

The nature of the work on the intensive care ward means that shared contact occurs between health professionals and patients; this inevitably means that transmission of resident and transient organisms from the hands of staff are more likely to occur unless strict attention is paid to effective infection control. Lack of appropriate education in applied microbiology appears to be hindering the provision of a safe environment in the intensive care unit.

The nurses' perception of the problem of hospital-acquired infection and the importance of microbiology will be influenced by knowledge of the scale of the problem within their own wards and units. This knowledge is vital in order to motivate an individual's application of appropriate knowledge to effective nursing practice. Nurses should be conscious of their present ability and responsibility to influence changes in attitudes of the health care team towards effective research-based infection-control practices. As technology advances and threatens to dominate the intensive care unit, nurses should seek clear definitions of their nursing role. The conclusions reached by the research project in question point towards the responsibility for infection control being placed within the nurses' remit. Other issues that fall directly in the realm and responsibility of nursing care and for which there are current difficulties in the provision of core standards are patient nutrition, pressure area care, wound care, patient safety and communication. The question that might be posed is: 'What is a nurse and what is nursing if we are failing to deliver the most basic standards of care?' Motivation is the result of internal and external factors. Internal motivators can be influenced, but not controlled, while external motivators can be created and controlled by others. In order to understand, predict and influence the motivation of individuals and groups, knowledge of theories of motivation provide an insight into the motivating process.

Nurses could have a much greater role to play in preventing hospital-acquired infection. The nurse is in constant contact with the patient and is normally the co-ordinator of care and of clinical information. The critically ill patient is temporarily placed in a vulnerable condition, unable to meet his or her own health needs. The intensive care nurse, in close proximity to the patient and providing individualized continuous care, is well placed to act as advocate to the patient. To adopt this role nurses must be educated, motivated and allowed to assist patients in transcending any barrier to having their needs met while they are undergoing health care (Witts 1992). By defining the health needs of the patient, and researching the contributions

of nursing, nurses will move forward, stating effectively what it is they do and why it makes a difference in the care of the critically ill patient.


## Hygiene compliance

The current low levels of compliance with recommended infection control in the intensive care unit are alarming. At the very least, acquired infections complicate a patient's recovery, increase discomfort and prolong hospital stay. At worst, they are a major contributory factor causing death in critically ill patients. In all cases, hospital-acquired infection reduces quality of care, quality of recovery and has possible consequences for the patient's present and future quality of life. Infection control is too often regarded as an optional extra of care. There was a need to effect change in clinical-infection-control practice while at the same time developing a quality-assurance system that embraced current research and sought to link infection-control behaviour to patient outcome and resource usage.

An evaluation of the effectiveness of infection-control care needs to be explicit within care processes. The rising need for clinical governance, demands quality in the NHS, global issues of antibiotic resistance, the increasing costs of health care, the theory-practice gap, the involvement of consumers and their rights, demonstration of high quality care and the economics of quality care. Researchers have highlighted this issue. Media attention on hospital infection rises and falls. The question posed is why we cannot use current information to support practice developments. A system that is focused on outcomes, where there is risk-factor assessment and process and one that is incorporated within a practical, cost-effective system, which enjoyed a high impact on behaviour, would seem to be favoured in the short-term and could be integrated within hospital information systems.


## Clinical governance in infection control

Risk management, clinical audit and demonstrating evidence of best practice in relation to infection control would seem to be essential components of raising the quality of caring for patients, which would, if managed effectively, improve information systems and potentially reduce the cost of health care. It will become increasingly important to examine the provision of health services and include some indication of patient outcome in relation to hospital-acquired infection as a necessary component of clinical audit.

## Prioritization of resources and infection control activity

Patients requiring intensive therapy are at a high risk of infection, and many of these infections are caused by poor techniques and are preventable. Work in an intensive care unit places high emotional, physical and professional demands on nurses. There is a multiplicity of intrinsic and extrinsic factors affecting the nurse working in the intensive care unit. These, in turn, influence perception of the problem of hospital-acquired infection. Because attitudes and values are learnt, they have the potential to be influenced, often in an automatic, unconscious fashion. As a result, strategies for improving clinical practice can be directed towards cognitive and behavioural components of individuals working in the intensive care unit. Problems of infection control in the intensive care unit should be analysed using a pragmatic approach, having first gained some understanding of the theories of individual and organizational behaviour. The social sciences can provide a framework to allow an understanding of human behaviour and these theories can be applied to the present arrangements for the fight against infection in the intensive care unit.

## Clarity of roles, responsibility and accountability for effective infection control

The nurse, in close proximity to the patient, is ideally placed to adopt a primary role in preventing infection. If nurses do not possess an adequate knowledge of the principles of microbiology or infection control, or do not apply this knowledge in clinical practice, and the culture of the organization is such that it inhibits creativity or enquiry, the knowledge for effective prevention of infection remains in the hands of a minority of specialists. If nurses can accept that hospital-acquired infection in British hospitals can be reduced by improving clinical practice, this means accepting the care we give is less than optimal. It then becomes the nurse's responsibility to become a guardian of the patient's microbial environment. In the light of current research indicating the risks of hospital-acquired infection to patients, there is a need for every patient admitted to have their infection status assessed and appropriate action taken. The control of infection is a responsibility shared by all disciplines working in the NHS, although, as a result of their regular hands-on contact with patients, nurses stand in the front line. In order to identify the need to advance personal knowledge of effective infection control, when social pressures to maintain the present status quo are high, the nurse must be aware of the importance of acquiring a sound knowledge of patient needs and applying the principles of microbiology in nursing practice to all stages of the nursing process documentation.

Infection control is generally taught as microbiology and not infection control as applied to practice. Nursing lecturers find infection control difficult to teach, and nursing students find it difficult to learn. It would appear that the teaching and learning styles being used are not conducive to the effective uptake of information and transfer of knowledge. There are barriers to implementing effective infection-control practice, and researchers have effectively shown that key elements of motivation are intrinsic to effective infection control but that health care professionals show resistance to educational programmes. There is a need for the biological sciences to be taught as core subjects in the education of nurses in order that they practise nursing care efficiently and effectively. The most powerful change that could affect standards of infection control is that of nursing-practice development in infection control. This requires changes in health professionals, services and organizations. Considering the increasing pressures on nurses – high workloads, reduced staffing and low morale – further practice developments need to be facilitated and monitored through a central process involving experts from clinical practice, audit, infection control, education, research and change management.

> The ultimate challenge is to develop an empirical basis for choosing interventions in the face of specific barriers to evidence-based practice, requiring both quantitative and qualitative methods to judge . . . not just the effectiveness of interventions, but gain an understanding of the process of professional behaviour change, and greater insight is needed into the personal skills and attributes that influence the effectiveness of individuals involved in changing behaviour (NHS Centre for Reviews and Dissemination 1999).

# References

Hope K (1998) Starting out with action research. Revisited Nurse Researcher 6(2): 16-26.

Inglis TJJI, Sproat LJ, Hawkey PM et al. (1992a) Infection control in intensive care units: national survey. British Journal of Anaesthesia 68(3):216-220.

Inglis TJJI, Sproat, LJ, Sherratt MJ et al. (1992b) Gastro-duodenal dysfunction as a cause of gastric bacterial overgrowth in patients undergoing mechanical ventilation of the lungs. British Journal of Anaesthesia 68(6):499-502.

Inglis TJJI, Sherratt MJ, Sproat LJ et al. (1993) Gastro-duodenal dysfunctional and bacterial colonisation of the ventilated lung. Lancet 341(2): 10.

McCormack B (1999a) Managing Practice Development. Practice Development Symposium – Foundation for Nursing Studies Practice Development Forum. Blackpool, 4-5 March 1999.

McCormack B (1999b) Evidence, Context and Facilitation: a model for implementing research into practice use. Practice Development Symposium – Foundation for Nursing Studies Practice Development Forum. Blackpool, 4-5 March 1999.

NHS Centre for Reviews and Dissemination (1999) Effective health care: getting evidence into practice. Effective Health Care Bulletin. The University of York, (February) 5(1): 1-16.

Sproat LJ, Inglis TJJI (1992) Preventing infection in the intensive care unit: a systematic approach to a standardisation of care. British Journal of Intensive Care (September) 2(6): 275-285.

Titchen A (1999) A conceptual framework for supporting practice development. Practice Development Symposium – Foundation for Nursing Studies Practice Development Forum. Blackpool, 4-5 March 1999.

Waterman H (1994) Meaning of Visual Impairment: developing ophthalmic nursing care. Manchester: University of Manchester.

Witts P (1992) Patient advocacy in nursing. In Kenworthy N, Chambers I (eds.) Themes and Perspectives in Nursing. Edinburgh: Churchill Livingstone.

# CHAPTER FOUR
# Grounded theory

MARK LIMB

## Introduction

Trying to grasp an understanding of the practical application of qualitative research procedures can be daunting for academics, health care professionals and students. The philosophical underpinnings and complex procedures used can often serve to baffle and confuse those undertaking such studies in the early stages of their research careers.

This chapter has been written to identify the issues related to the use of grounded theory in practice. The work describes the processes undertaken while investigating the experiences of adult individuals undergoing limb-reconstruction procedures in a large inner-city teaching hospital.

## Prior to the study

One of the most important things to note about any research project is that it needs contextualizing. This can be done in two ways. The first is by providing a background and setting for the research, thus giving the reader an insight into the origins of the work and some idea of its generalizability or use to them within their own field of practice. The second is by providing a review of the literature that identifies the state of knowledge relating to the subject matter at the beginning of the research; this can later be used to consider how the research undertaken has added to the body of literature available to health care practitioners.

The introduction, background and literature review are therefore considered very important parts of the research process. They serve to set the scene for the research and identify/justify the need for the study. In fact, with reference to the literature, some authors believe that reviewing and evaluating such is central to the research process. Its purpose, according to Cormack and Benton (1996), is to produce a summary of previous work that should clearly describe the extent of the current knowledge base. Gaps in the knowledge base or inconsistencies both in terms of the research results and in the theoretical frameworks should be restated succinctly, thus forming the rationale for conducting further research.

However, the author intended that the research to be undertaken would be fundamentally qualitative in nature and various other authors note problems in reviewing the literature prior to such a study taking place. Benton (1996) states that at the early stages of such a study an in-depth critique of the literature might provide a framework that includes categories that are inappropriate or incomplete. In addition, Morse (1994) feels that knowledge is a possible contaminant, a possible source of bias and a threat to validity. However, the author believes that such views do not account for literature that may have been previously read by himself, or prior experience obtained; it would be impossible to remove this from memory. Strauss and Corbin (1990) would describe such as 'theoretical sensitivity', which they define as 'a personal quality of the researcher. It indicates an awareness of the subtleties of the meaning of data'. They point out that it can come from a variety of sources, mainly: literature, professional experience and personal experience. They also point out that it can be a stimulus for the research question as it points to relatively unexplored areas, suggests need for further development or highlights contradictions or ambiguities. DePoy and Gitlin (1993) further point out that researchers undertaking qualitative research may review the literature before conducting the research to confirm the need for such an approach to be taken. As such, there is an argument that it is not an absolute requirement that a literature review should not be undertaken prior to a qualitative study. What is perhaps more important is that the researcher makes explicit to the reader the theoretical sensitivity being brought into the study. They can then decide whether or not the study has been biased as a result of this. The first task, therefore, was to make this explicit, and this was done using the elements of theoretical sensitivity as identified by Strauss and Corbin (1990). For these writers, theoretical sensitivity is categorized into three broad areas (and the researcher made initial notes on such in order to give the reader insight into the knowledge and experience being carried into the study):

1. **Personal experience**: With reference to the concepts of external fixation and limb reconstruction, the author had no personal experience to write about.
2. **Professional experience**: The researcher had a good deal of experience here. Summarizing this was very useful as it provided a thorough description of involvement in care and practice to date. Reflection on professional experience and patient-care episodes was undertaken, and the author was able to reach the conclusion that many psychosocial

issues were being experienced by patients but there was little done in practice to help the individuals come to terms with their changing appearance and roles. It was useful to make this explicit, as it gave the reader an insight into what can be fundamentally regarded as the background to the study.

3. **The Literature**: This can be divided into the following two areas:

    Technical literature: journal articles and books, and to summarize these the author wrote a literature review of all such reading up to the point of the study. Having done this, it was concluded that there was very little research exploring the psychosocial issues relating to limb reconstruction and that most of the published research was quantitative in nature and had a medical direction or focus. This therefore justified the need for a study, and writing and reporting the results of the literature review would give any potential reader an insight into the potential influences this may have had on the research outcomes.

    Non-technical literature: newspaper reports and television programmes. Again, a review of any such material read and seen by the researcher was made in order to set before the reader any insights that could potentially bias or influence the study.

In order to make the potential bias of the theoretical sensitivity more evident, the author then constructed a preliminary conceptual framework. Having said that the research intended to use grounded theory as the primary research method, there is a good deal of argument within the literature to suggest that a framework is not required in order to conduct the study; in fact, it could be regarded as detrimental. Benton (1996) points out that the researcher should approach data collection without a preconceived framework. Without the open-minded approach, he feels there is a danger that significant material may be ignored since data that are not seen as fitting the existing model may be disregarded. However, Miles and Huberman (1994) feel that something is already known about the phenomenon but not enough to house a theory. They also point out that the researcher has an idea of the parts of the phenomenon that are not well understood but knows:

a) where to look for these things
b) in which settings
c) among which actors
d) how to gather information

Bearing these things in mind, they argue that at the outset one usually has at least a rudimentary conceptual framework, a set of general research questions, some notions about sampling and some initial ideas about data-gathering devices. The advice of Stratton (1996) is that the researcher should make the theoretical base explicit and then interview and code based on this. In doing this, the researcher also acknowledges the view of Marshall and Rossman (1995), who feel that in examining a specific setting or set of individuals the researcher should show how the case of a larger phenomenon is being studied. By linking the specific research questions to larger theoretical constructs, the writer shows that the particulars of the study serve to illuminate larger issues and, therefore, are of significance. The advice is to develop a conceptual framework for the study that is thorough, concise and elegant.

For the purpose of this study, the conceptual framework presented in Figure 4.1 below was developed to reflect the theoretical sensitivity that the researcher was bringing to the study.

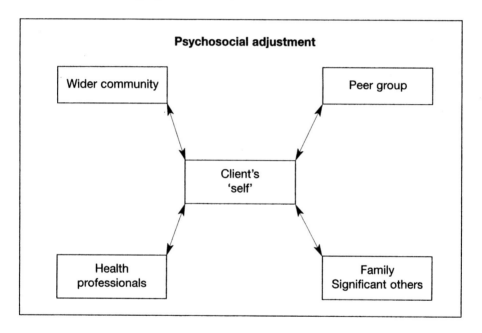

**Figure 4.1** The preliminary conceptual framework.

# Figure 4.1 explained

### Definition of terms

Definitions are based upon the professional and theoretical sensitivity of the researcher.

**The client's self** is the participants' view of how they see themselves since having had an external fixation device in situ. This view of the self has to be regarded as being both descriptive and evaluative. It is acknowledged that the 'self' aspect of the participant is influenced by a number of other factors out of their control. These factors exist within **the environment**. This is defined, for the purpose of this research, as any context in which the participants may find themselves. Within this environment, the participants will come into contact with a wide variety of individuals. For the purpose of this research, these were separated into groups as the author intends to examine if these different groups affect, or are perceived to affect, the self-concept in different ways.

**Health professionals** are often the first to come into contact with the clients. Post-operatively, these can be nurses, doctors, physiotherapists and occupational therapists.

**Family and significant others** are often the next to have close contact with the clients. They may be less familiar with such devices, and reactions may be different. For the purpose of this research, partners, parents, siblings and the participants' own children would fall into this category.

**The peer group** is seen as being made up of individuals who may come into regular close contact with the participants such as friends, work colleagues, fellow students etc.

**The wider community** is regarded as the individuals with whom the participants may come into contact in a variety of situations; however, there would have been no previous contact, or any intended further contact, with such.

The researcher also intends to explore how these interactions between the participants and other individuals affect the participants' **behaviour**, such is regarded as any response to the actual or perceived attitudes/actions towards the participants.

## The study aims

Like quantitative studies, qualitative studies also need aims; though, as Holloway and Wheeler (1996) point out, these should be less directional than those of a quantitative nature. The following aims were identified from the above framework:

- to examine the experience of the clients once discharged from hospital
- to identify how they feel the surgery has affected their sense of self
- to examine how others in the environment are perceived to act/react towards the clients
- to examine how the clients deal with their feelings regarding these perceptions

- to provide health care professionals with an evidence base for practice that can help enhance the experience of the client.

## Methodology

The methodology of grounded theory was first described by Glaser and Strauss (1967). Its theoretical framework is derived from the symbolic interactionist school of social-psychology (Mead 1934, Blumer 1969), which Holloway and Wheeler (1996) point out focuses on the process of inter-action, exploring human behaviour and social rules. Chenitz and Swanson (1986) feel that the reality or meaning of the situation is created by people and leads to action and the consequences of action. Implicit and explicit in these descriptions is the notion that people are reacting to particular cir-cumstances. However, the reactivity to situations in itself could be regarded as simplistic. There is much more to interaction than reaction. Morse (1994) points out that individuals order their world by engaging in a process of negotiation and re-negotiation by making reflexive use of sym-bols and by interpreting and eliciting meaning in situations rather than by simply reacting. In accepting the symbolic interactionist perspective, the researcher accepted the model of the person as active and creative rather than passive, and as existing in a reality that is fluid and constantly created and modified. This seemed to reflect well the desire of the author to exam-ine the self in relation to others within the environment and to try and elucidate the thought processes of individuals when faced with the cir-cumstances set before them as they come into contact with any variety of given individuals and contexts.

Morse further adds that the methodology is process-orientated and therefore not just a description of values and beliefs. It allows for changes over time and identifies stages and phases that the individual undergoes and therefore seemed congruent with the research aims of exploring the changes in self-concept over time. The particular goal is to explore the social processes that occur in human interaction and to discover theoreti-cally complete explanations about particular phenomena.

However, the researcher had to acknowledge that life is a complex situ-ation for these individuals that undergo limb reconstruction as they enter and exit a number of different environmental situations in the treatment history. This results in multiple changes in appearance as a number of tech-niques are put to use on their affected limbs. However, Chenitz and Swanson (1986) feel that grounded theory is particularly useful for describ-ing behaviour in such complex situations. In addition, Morse (1994) feels that it is useful for eliciting and describing the psychological and social processes that have been developed by people to make sense of their world.

If described, these processes can then be used to enable others in similar situations to make sense of their actions and reasoning used in everyday coping after surgery.

## Sampling

Sandelowski (1986) points out that representativeness in qualitative research concerns the data and not the sampling units. In effect, it is not bound by positivistic parameters and uses non-probability sampling procedures. Weiner and Wysmans (1990) feel that this is not done in terms of individuals or units of time but in terms of concepts, dimensions and variations. What seems to be of particular importance here is the experience of the clients and their ability to be able to provide information relating to concept development. Therefore, individuals need to be selected based upon their ability to provide information not via random selection; such positivist procedures may eliminate those with necessary experience from the sample resulting in data that are weak and limited in terms of analytic potential. Miles and Huberman (1994) further support this in documenting that it is not representativeness that is a concern; in fact, what is required are informants, episodes and interactions that are being driven by a conceptual question. As Morse and Field (1996) point out, the purpose of qualitative research is to discover meaning not measure the distribution of attributes within a population. Any client with sufficient time post-operatively will have developed coping strategies that would be of interest to the researcher, and it was therefore decided to select any clients able to give informed consent with at least three months post-discharge time to discuss their experiences.

With specific reference to numbers to be included, one of the problems was how many this should be, and the literature regarding this seemed to be somewhat confusing to the researcher. Swanson (1986) identifies the number as between 20 and 50, which the researcher felt too large, particularly as there were only approximately 60 participants at any one time from which selection could be made. However, Stern (1993) points out that nurse researchers with little experience between the years of 1967 and 1987 frequently invented rigid rules that broke the true canons of creativity inherent within the original philosophy of grounded theory, one of these being that to include fewer than 12 participants is unacceptable.

Other researchers have tried to ascertain the numbers by analysing the characteristics of the population. Kuzel (1992) feels that the following types of population need the stated numbers:

Homogeneous 6–8
Heterogeneous 12–20

In essence, the researcher felt that this particular population was fairly homogeneous in that the group were all undergoing similar treatment processes; though one does have to acknowledge that this would be for a variety of reasons. However, the researcher felt justified in defining this as a homogeneous group in terms of limb reconstruction, as opposed, for example, to examining the self-concept of a group consisting of persons undergoing a variety of treatment interventions (that is reconstructive facial surgery, enterostomal surgery and reconstructive breast surgery). Such would be regarded as more heterogeneous and requiring larger samples in order to be able to accommodate the variety of experiences inherent within such a population.

One of the most important aspects of sampling in grounded theory is the notion that this should be done theoretically. Morse and Field (1996) define theoretical sampling as sampling on the basis of what has been learned from previous data sources. In effect, individuals were chosen as needed and not before the study began.

## The sample

The researcher attended the outpatient clinic on a weekly basis over a period of one year. Following discussion with the consultant and the clinical nurse specialist, potential patients were identified for inclusion in the study. If the participants were still willing to be involved, they were introduced to the researcher who gave them a further overview of the project and its aims and objectives. In this discussion the consent form and information sheet were discussed in order that any potential problems and/or misunderstandings could be clarified.

Each participant had a very specific history; some had been undergoing treatment in other institutions for many years prior to their present therapy, and the limb-reconstruction unit is a relatively close-knit environment where many of the clients discuss their histories and compare and contrast their lifestyles. These factors were the cause of a great deal of anxiety for the researcher for, while each individual had a wealth of personal characteristics and attributes which the researcher would like to use to describe the population, there was the possibility that if this were to be done the participants would be very easily identifiable. So it was decided for the purpose of this study that sample details would be presented in two ways:

1. **specific biographical data** about individuals from which those persons could not be identified, for example age, gender and type of frame
2. **general data** about the whole of the sample

This gives the reader an insight into the experience that the research participants were bringing to the situation and gives an awareness of such things as the reasons the individuals were having limb reconstruction, previous medical interventions and their family and social support networks. Over the one-year time period that the study took place, seven participants were selected for inclusion.

## Constant comparison and saturation

While the stages of data collection and analysis in the following section are described separately, it is important that the reader understands that these occur simultaneously. Constant comparison is one of the most important and fundamental canons of grounded theory that should not be compromised. It is insufficient to collect all the data from all of the participants then analyse them. What one finds in the first interview drives data collection from the second. The findings from both the first and second drive what is collected from the third and so on. Holloway and Wheeler (1996) feel that this helps increase the amount of data available and helps develop the categories and concepts identified from the interview transcripts that can be included in the developing theory.

This leads on to the notion of saturation. Saturation of the codes is an important issue in this particular methodology. Benton (1996) states that a category can be said to be saturated when examination of the data reveals no new properties and the categories are completely developed. If this is not achieved, it leads to premature closure, which Wilson and Hutchinson (1996) feel occurs as the researcher fails to move beyond the face content in the narrative thus making categories be based purely on participants' descriptive phrases instead of concepts. Morse (1994) does, though, refer to the myth of saturation as she feels that if the researcher were to select another sample of people new ideas would be formed and the researcher may be faced with a dilemma. However, in this instance, the researcher chose to select only individuals from one particular group and did not feel that the issue would arise in this instance.

## Data collection

The best way of finding out how people think, feel or behave is simply to ask them about it (Cormack 1984), and Stern et al. (1982) feel that the dynamic psychosocial and social processes that are the focus of grounded theory may be observed from social interaction and listening to what informants say about themselves. It is therefore clear that the interview is an important form of data collection in grounded theory.

It was decided that unstructured interviews would be the most appropriate way to collect data for the purpose of this study. Unstructured interviews are interviews that carry no predetermined format. Grbich (1999) refers to them as guided, and Porter (1996) as in-depth. Importantly, Porter refers to the notion of power within this type of interview. While the semi- and unstructured interview formats carry a degree of researcher control, this particular type carries less influence on the part of the interviewer and more influence on the part of the interviewee. Burns and Grove (1987) feel that these interviews are important in discovering what problems exist in a social scene and how the people involved handle them, this notion being highly congruent with the philosophy of grounded theory and the aims of the research.

Polit and Hungler (1995) feel that an unstructured interview is one in which the researcher proceeds with no preconceived view of the content or the flow of the information to be gathered. Burns and Grove (1987) further add that the researcher is to remain open-minded about what will be found. However, May (1991) feels that it is misleading to say there are no preconceived ideas. She feels it would be difficult to approach any interviews as a neutral element. Holloway and Wheeler (1996) further add that researchers have their own agenda, that they have some idea of interest in mind at the outset and the goal is to discover and understand the informant's perspective. As such, Swanson (1986) advises the use of a guide containing a brief set of questions, a topical outline or a major theme to discuss. Holloway and Wheeler (1996) refer to this as an aide-memoire; however, they do stipulate that there should be no predetermined questions, as suggested by Swanson (1986), as this would add unnecessary structure to the interview and limit the potential range of responses that may be obtained from, for example, a topical or thematic approach to the interview.

Initial interviews took place using themes from the preliminary conceptual framework as a guide. Time was taken to allow the participants to talk about their experiences when coming into contact with given individuals/groups in the contexts in which the participant interacted. Participants were interviewed for approximately one hour in their own homes. This served two purposes: first of all, it put them in the position of power: they were in their own environment and this would give them a greater sense of control. The researcher was the visitor in this instance, as opposed to the outpatient scenario whereby the participants are subsumed under the health care system. Secondly, as a result of this, the participants would be more at ease and feel able to comfortably express themselves as individuals and not as patients. This would mean that the interviews would more likely be about personal issues as opposed to physiological and biomechanical issues, which are often the focus of the outpatient interaction.

Initially, the interviews took place relating to the original conceptual framework as identified previously. However, as the study progressed, the interviews became more structured and related to the clarification of ideas developed from the interviews with previous participants. Finally, all interviews were tape recorded and then transcribed by the researcher.

# Data analysis and coding

## Open coding

The first stage in data analysis, as identified by Strauss and Corbin (1990), is referred to as open coding. This has been further divided by some authors into level one and level two coding (Streubert and Carpenter 1995, Silverman 1993), the aims as identified by the latter are to develop categories that illuminate the data and then saturate them with many appropriate cases.

Level one coding is the first stage. This is sometimes referred to as substantive coding because the researcher attempts to codify the substance of the data. Strauss and Corbin (1990) identify that this can be done in three ways:

1. code the entire document
2. code sentences or paragraphs
3. code the data line by line

Benton (1996) and Glaser and Strauss (1967) advise that each sentence/incident should be coded into as many substantive codes as possible. However, this could prove confusing and time-consuming, and Miles and Huberman (1994) feel that it is much more appropriate to assign the single most appropriate (more encompassing) code amongst those related to the given research question. They further feel that the researcher should be clear about what constitutes a unit of analysis and feel that a sentence or multi-sentence chunk is better. This would seem sensible bearing in mind that the researcher is trying to identify the context in which events occur (Strauss and Corbin 1990), in which case this would be more identifiable from multi-sentence chunks than discrete actions selected from the transcript.

Streubert and Carpenter (1995) feel that in substantive coding the labels applied to the data should either be words used by the participant or constructed by the researcher. Hutchinson (1986), on the other hand, feels that they should be relatively simple words as used by the participant. Whichever the researcher chooses, though, they are referred to by Strauss (1987) as *in vivo* codes and as such should reflect the reality of the participant. There is here the potential for conflicts in emphasis of thinking as the researcher may try to force labels onto the data. Glaser and Strauss (1967) advise that in such cases the researcher should stop, write a memo that provides an illustration of the idea and then assign a relevant code.

To clarify this issue, one can refer to the work of Clarke (1992), who points out problems with coding. He feels that the same word may have different connotations in different circumstances. Here he is obviously referring to the everyday vernacular that is evident in discourse. However, we should not see this as a difficulty. Schutz (1962) sees this as a treasure house of ready-made preconstituted types and characteristics all socially derived and carrying an open horizon of unexplored content. While similar words may have different meanings, it is not acceptable to reject their use based purely upon this factor. Cicourel (1973) feels that the everyday vernacular requires a context to determine the meaning of a person's discourse. Therefore, to locate its meaning, simply supply the context. So, while the same word may have different meanings in different circumstances, the researcher simply has to supply the context of the circumstances in order to be able to fully appreciate its meaning. While in the process of open coding, this may be difficult; when axial (level three) coding is undertaken, the context becomes much more important.

After undertaking and transcribing three initial interviews, the job of the researcher was to begin the process of open coding. Attempts were first made to code the entire document, and, having read through the transcript of interview 1, the author decided that this could be labelled as follows:

**Covering up:** based on the idea that the participant seemed to be taking steps to hide the frame and their apparent disability.

However, the researcher felt that this needed breaking down further and decided to take the paragraph-by-paragraph approach and then came up with the following labels:

**Shock:** based on the client's surprise at the initial appearance of the frame.

'I think it distressed me seeing my leg in such a bad way, I don't know ... it was horrible.'

**Recuperating:** based on the client's desire to get physically well.

'I didn't go out for the first few months . . . partly because I was trying to recuperate.'

**Covering up the fixator:** based on the client's desire to prevent others from seeing the frame.

> 'I quite enjoy wearing skirts; it's more feminine. But . . . it's the only way to cover up the frame.'

**Covering up the disability:** based on the client's desire not to be seen as physically disabled.

> 'I never went out in the wheelchair . . . because it attracted more attention I suppose . . . I like people to know that I can get about.'

These broad labels were then used to start gathering data from subsequent interviewees, and, after open coding of each one of these on a paragraph-by-paragraph basis, the labels identified in Table 4.1 were applied to the experiences of the participants.

**Table 4.1** Open coding using the paragraph-by-paragraph approach

| Number 1 | Number 2 | Number 3 |
| --- | --- | --- |
| shock | shock | shock |
| recuperating | recovering | relying on others |
| covering fixator | covering fixator | covering fixator |
| covering disability | covering disability | rejecting disability |
| | objectification | rejecting objectification |
| | protecting the limb | |

The author, at this point, began to reflect on these two approaches to coding and felt that to code whole documents and/or paragraphs may be self-limiting. Consideration was given to the notion that one may be only looking for what one could see, or only seeing things that one knew were there (for instance as a result of inherent theoretical sensitivity). The author therefore decided to recode the whole of the three transcripts using the sentence-by-sentence approach and came up with the labels identified in Table 4.2.

This exercise gave a much richer list of labels and identified a much wider range of phenomena. It seems that analysis was moving from a description of how things appeared to reflect more adequately what was happening. The sentence-by-sentence approach provided a great deal more insight than the paragraph, multisentence chunk or whole-document approach. The totality of the experience was much more visible as the researcher could not ignore any aspects of the interview transcript.

**Table 4.2** Open coding using the sentence-by-sentence approach

| Number 1 | Number 2 | Number 3 |
|---|---|---|
| shock | previous experience | surprise |
| being like others | misinformed | change in dress code |
| focusing on limb | being like others | comparing with others |
| staying in | changing clothing | comfort zones |
| being accepted | recovering | getting used to it |
| covering frame | being different | helplessness |
| perceptions of others | perceptions of others | loss of control |
| reactions of others | being like others | being a burden |
| changing presentation | hitting back | losing it |
| rationalizing | avoiding the public | in the public eye |
| ignoring advice | being known | interfering others |
| object of curiosity | objectification | does he take sugar? |
| recuperating | understanding others | coping |
| lacking confidence | normality | rejecting disability |
| maintaining control | shrugging off | rationalizing |
| seeking assurance | dressing differently | avoiding the gaze |
| fitting in | keeping occupied | being normal |
| avoiding others | relying on others | objectification |
| | interrogation | nosy parkers |
| | | perceptions of others |
| | | avoiding the public gaze |
| | | drawing attention |
| | | treading carefully |

A further four interviews were carried out. Again, these were done bearing in mind the notion of theoretical sampling, interviews built upon what had already been gathered and were used to develop appropriate categories. Table 4.3 shows the list of labels applied to the phenomena identified within the transcripts:

**Table 4.3** Open coding of interviews 4 to 7

| Number 4 | Number 5 | Number 6 | Number 7 |
|---|---|---|---|
| shock | regret | shock | becoming aware |
| protecting the limb | covering up | avoiding the public | avoiding the gaze |
| recuperating | objectification | objectification | recuperating |
| nosy parkers | nosy parkers | covering up | keeping out of the way |
| being mothered | being different | rejecting disability | objectification |
| covering up | covering up | relying on others | covering up |
| protecting the limb | avoiding the gaze | helplessness | becoming aware |

**Table 4.3**  Open coding of interviews 4 to 7 (contd)

| Number 4 | Number 5 | Number 6 | Number 7 |
|---|---|---|---|
| helplessness | being different | comfort zones | relying on others |
| drawing attention | avoiding stereotypes | accepting disability | |
| questioning | rejecting disability | ignoring others | |
| rejecting disability | attracting attention | | |
| accepting disability | | | |

As one can see from the number of labels applied to the transcripts, the interviews were becoming more focused, and the information asked of participants related to the issues brought up in previous interviews. A process of data collection was taking place in order that relevant information was obtained for the purpose of analysis.

In addition, the process of data reduction was also occurring. If one compares the number of labels applied to the transcripts, the following will be observed.

In interviews 1 to 3 (Table 4.2), the number of labels applied gradually increases as the researcher attempts to gain as many data as possible for the purpose of analysis. However, as the focus of the study is identified, the number of labels gradually decreases as clarity of purpose is achieved (see interviews 4 to 7: Table 4.3).

Having developed individual codes, the researcher then had to compare these and start to assign them to clusters and categories; this is sometimes referred to as level two coding (Streubert and Carpenter 1995). Grbich (1999) points out that this is not simply fracturing the data and grouping conceptually but focusing on the constant comparison of incidents. This prevents inappropriate labelling and conceptual forcing. This is important at this stage as Hutchinson (1986) points out that the categories are now being formulated by the researcher and may become more abstract. Clarke (1992) is further critical of this type of coding; she feels this may be used by propagandists to increase influence. However, in response to such an argument, to have true meaning a category must be capable of being uniquely defined. In theory, this has to come from the informants' descriptions of their experiences and the descriptions given must adequately fit into the categories as labelled. This is achieved through constant comparison and ensuring that as concepts emerge incident is compared with incident to ensure that they are appropriately labelled (Grbich 1999). Strauss and Corbin (1990) also advocate that the labels be checked with the participant to ensure that interpretation is appropriate; as such this does go some way to ensuring the theory reflects the reality of the participant and not the expectations of the researcher. In addition, during the process of theoretical sampling, one is highlighting and selecting concepts that are of relevance because of the discussion generated around them. However, in support of Corbin's notion, one does have to reiterate the problems associated with the suspending of personal values and beliefs and account for the fact that this may influence the theory as it develops. In fact, Wilson and Hutchinson (1996) feel that the importing of concepts will prevent the development of theoretical and conceptual codes and lead to under-analysis of the textual narrative data.

The following are lists of the categories that were used in the final theory with the relevant labels underneath, also included are notes made on my views of the relevance of the categories.

**Shock**
was made up of the labels:
shock, surprise, previous experience, misinformed, getting used to it, focusing on the limb, being like others, regret, becoming aware and comparing with others.

**Note:** this category seemed to relate to the first perceptions of the sight of the frame on recovery from the anaesthetic. The perceptions were based on and related to previous experience and the information provided by the consenting medical officer. Despite both there was often a sense of shock. Shock does not appear to be the prime phenomenon as this is a static label. While shock was experienced, the main focus was on **becoming aware** of the presence of the frame, and the context in which there were others with frames was important here. Therefore, the label for this category was changed accordingly.

**Getting over it**
was made up of the labels:
recuperating, recovering, helplessness, coping and staying in.

**Note:** this seems to be about getting physically fit post-operatively, and, during this phase, while the client is unwell there is no real concern over appearance.

**Keeping out of the way**
was made up of the labels:
avoiding questions, avoiding public situations, avoiding others and avoiding the gaze.

**Note:** this seems to be about clients not getting into situations in which they may feel objectified. This seems to occur when members of the public stare and ask questions about the fixator and their treatment history.

**Hiding it**
was made up of the labels:
covering up the frame, fitting in, dressing differently, change in dress code, changes in presentation, being different, changing clothing, being like others and being accepted.
   Note: this seems to be about dressing in such a way that the frame is less conspicuous but allowing, where possible, an expression of the self.

**Stepping out**
was made up of the labels:
ignoring advice, rejecting disability, does he take sugar?, interfering others, perceptions of others, being a burden, rejecting/accepting the disability, avoiding stereotypes, ignoring advice, hitting back, losing it and maintaining self-control.
   Note: this seems to relate to the clients' perceptions of how they feel others perceive them based upon their appearance. In response to their perceptions, they appear to reject certain symbols of disability. In addition, it also seems to be about responses to the way the clients are treated as mentally disabled by others.

**Objectification**
was made up of the labels:
object of curiosity, shrugging off, objectification, being different, comfort zones, being known, in the public eye, rejection of objectification, interrogation, nosy parkers, drawing attention, lacking confidence, understanding others, perceptions of others, drawing/attracting attention, questioning, being accepted and being normal.
   Note: this seems to be a very broad category about how the clients feel when other people stare at them and make them feel like freak shows. It seems to fit into a number of other categories, and this was clarified in further interviews. Many of the data could actually be recoded to fit other categories, especially 'covering up' and 'keeping out of the way'. This appeared to be the basis of an interlinking (core) category.

   As a result of constant comparison and data reduction, the following categories seemed to hold most theoretical relevance:

• becoming aware
• getting over it
• avoiding stares
• avoiding questions

- hiding it
- stepping out

# Expanding categorical properties and dimensions

At the same time as the above levels of analysis were taking place, the researcher was also trying to elicit data that served to expand the properties and dimensions of the categories (Strauss and Corbin 1990) (**properties** are the characteristics/attributes and **dimensions** are the location of that property along a continuum). Table 4.4 shows extracts from field notes that relate to the category 'hiding it':

**Table 4.4** Properties and dimensions of the category 'hiding it'

| Properties | Dimensions |
|---|---|
| Not letting family see it | 4 to 5 days |
| Extended family | Covered at first – gradually exposed |
| Going outside with frame visible | Wouldn't do it |
| Use of bag to cover frame | When outside |
| Curiosity vs. shock | Achieving balance |

After the process of expanding categorical properties and dimensions, the researcher's awareness of subtleties in data began to increase, and it was at this stage that the developed categories really started to become significant in terms of their meanings. However, the researcher still felt that he was still only coding what could be seen in the data and felt that greater analytic depth was required in order that relevant and in-depth theory could be generated. In order that **theoretical sensitivity** can be developed further, Strauss and Corbin (1990) advocate the use of the following basic questions to be asked of the phenomena in each category:

- Who?
- When?
- Where?
- What?
- How?
- How much?
- Why?

Table 4.5 highlights a selection of field notes. Again, examples from the category 'hiding it' are cited. The ideas presented here reflect a situation where a participant was made to feel abnormal by the inconsiderate stares of people walking past as he was resting during a walk.

**Table 4.5** Properties and dimensions of the category 'hiding it'

| Who? | onlookers |
|------|-----------|
| When? | at first |
| Where? | outside |
| What? | showing them |
| How? | used to allow them to see it |
| How much? | freely at first but not any more |
| Why? | they think 'He's not a normal person' |

A summary of ideas identified in the whole of the transcripts relating to this category is presented in Table 4.6 below. The wide range of information comes from conducting interviews with the questions to enhance theoretical sensitivity identified above and applying the important principle of constant comparison at all times.

**Table 4.6** Summary of ideas brought together for the category 'hiding it'

| Why hide it? | prevent staring |
|--------------|-----------------|
| | prevent cold |
| | general reactions of others |
| | what people might say/think |
| | prevent offence to others |
| From whom? | pedestrians |
| | shoppers |
| | customers |
| | people walking |
| | patients and relatives |
| Where? | on the street |
| | in shops |
| | in pubs |
| | in restaurants |
| | at college |
| | in hospital |
| When? | out shopping |
| | out walking |
| | out for a meal |
| | outpatient visit |
| Feelings experienced? | hatred of leggings |
| | it's ugly |
| | unfeminine |
| | ugly |
| | don't have words |
| | not bothered |

**Table 4.6** Summary of ideas brought together for the category 'hiding it' (contd)

| What did they do? | cover with bandage |
| | plan what to wear |
| | wear long skirts |
| | don't show anyone |
| | dress from waist up |
| | use bag/blanket |
| | don't cover it at all |
| Consequences of what they did | feels more feminine |
| | fit in more |
| | people not shocked |
| | prevents stereotypes |
| | prevents offence |
| | prevents family distress |
| | feel part of family |

The above exercise was undertaken with all categories on each interview. One can see from the above that a great deal of good-quality data can be generated by bearing in mind the questions advised for increasing theoretical sensitivity.

# Axial coding

Originally, open coding had helped the researcher to break the data down into discrete parts; these were labelled using the words of the participants and words that the researcher felt appropriate. The additional questions asked to increase theoretical sensitivity further helped the researcher to clarify that the labels were appropriate and that the categorization of these labels was relevant.

The next stage of data analysis is referred to by Strauss and Corbin (1990) as 'axial coding'. Streubert and Carpenter (1995) refer to this as 'level three coding'. They suggest that the researcher now asks the following questions:

- What is going on in the data?
- What is the focus of the study and the relationship of the data to the study?
- What is the problem being dealt with?
- What process is helping the participant cope with the problem?

Effectively, what the researcher is trying to ascertain here are the basic sociopsychological processes as they continue over time regardless of varying conditions (Glaser 1978). Strauss and Corbin (1990) suggest that the questions as identified in Figure 4.2 are asked which help to identify relationships amongst the categories. These are presented in the form of the paradigm.

---

The **conditions** that give rise to the phenomena.

The **context** in which it is embedded.

The **actional/interactional** strategies by which it is managed.

The **consequences** of those strategies.

The **intervening conditions** that influence the situation.

---

**Figure 4.2** The paradigm.

Hutchinson (1986) points out that this begins to link the data together in a new form, the number of categories is further reduced and major new categories are generated. These are based on the analyst's knowledge of nursing and academic experience and are referred to as theoretical/conceptual codes as opposed to the *in vivo* or substantive codes that the analyst developed early on (Wilson and Hutchinson 1996).

The model in Figure 4.2 presented above is written in a fairly simplistic style. However, in reality, it was often quite difficult to apply it to the categories. This tended to be more so where the data lacked depth or quality. However, subsequent interviews were used to gather data to enable more thorough application.

In addition, it was often quite confusing as to which part of the paradigm a category fitted. For example 'avoiding stares' could, out of context, be regarded as an action to prevent the participant seeing people stare: they look at the floor so that they do not see others looking at them. However, it could also be seen as a consequence of people staring. Such problems were overcome by sampling the data to establish their exact position in the model. The following example highlights avoiding the gaze explicitly as an intentional action; however, some questioning revealed all was not as it seemed. One particular participant had originally said that he looked at the floor to be able to see where he was going; on probing further, a different reason for his action emerges.

A: You know people are looking at you, but you don't have to look back. If they're not staring, they can't ask you questions.

Q: So part of looking at the floor is not only about looking where you're going, it's also about not seeing other people's reactions?

A: Yes.

The problems regarding the position of categories within the paradigm were overcome by careful sampling of the data to determine the most relevant location. Again, where the data lacked depth, the researcher was able to focus subsequent interviews on appropriate issues so that theoretically relevant data could be obtained thus enabling the development of a theory that is grounded in the data. Figure 4.3 gives an example of the paradigm as applied to the category of 'hiding it'.

---

**Causal conditions**

People staring

People looking


**Phenomena**

Don't like public places


**Properties**

Inspect it

Give advice

Looking

Fixator

Fixator


**Dimensions**

That's what they do

They try to

They shouldn't be

They've never seen them before

Too big to cover


**Context**

In places where the participant feels that he is becoming an object of curiosity to others


**Actional/interactional strategies**

Bandage my leg over


**Intervening conditions**

Frame too large to cover with conventional bag or expanded trousers


**Consequences**

If it's covered, it doesn't look that bad really

---

**Figure 4.3** The paradigm as used in the category 'hiding it'.

The exercise of axial coding was very useful in restructuring the data the researcher had obtained. It also started to spark ideas about how the categories could be related to each other. While the category 'objectification', where the onlooker treated the participant almost as an object, had been re-allocated to a number of other categories, it now became more evident that this could be the interlinking category and potentially the core category: many of the phenomena related to this sense of objectification. Further analysis even demonstrated that the clients were suffering a sense of deviance and felt stigmatized as a result of the appearance. Investigation into the concepts of stigma and deviance demonstrated that this sense of self is suffered by many who have mutilating surgery and have dramatic changes in physical appearance. The analysis had therefore led the researcher to thinking about the types of literature that needed consideration in order to be able to examine the concepts that had been identified and develop them further. An example of one particular work that the researcher stared to read was Goffman (1963), his work on stigma helped to give consideration as to how appearance and disability may lead to judgements by others and feelings of inadequacy on the part of the judged.

## Core category

The development of a core category should follow axial coding (Strauss and Corbin 1990). The core category is defined by Benton (1996) as the category at the centre of the theory and should be capable of explaining much of the variation in behaviour discovered in the data. Most of the other categories and their properties should relate to the core category. Holloway and Wheeler (1996) point out that this is done by the process of selective coding whereby categories that do not fit within the theory are excluded from the overall explanation given for the particular phenomenon identified.

Strauss (1987) identifies six characteristics of the core category as:

- it recurs frequently
- it links the data together
- because it is central, it explains variation
- it has implications for formal/general theory
- as it becomes more detailed, theory moves forwards
- it permits maximum variation and analysis

On sampling the data for the paradigm such phenomena, or related phenomena, seemed to occur frequently. The core category seemed, therefore, to be about deviance and coming to terms with it and its effect on the participants' lifestyle. Coping with deviance seemed to be the essence of the study. The core category is presented in Figure 4.4 in terms of the requirements of the paradigm.

## Redefinition of the categorical labels

After further review of the categories and their content, the researcher looked again at the notion of abstraction of the categories. The labels in

**Phenomenon:**
sense of deviance

**Causal conditions:**
appearance
disability
people staring
people asking questions

| Properties: | Dimensions: | |
|---|---|---|
| familiarity with others | familiar | unfamiliar |
| personal feelings | bothered | not bothered |
| | mad | understanding |
| perceptions of normal | unscarred | disfigured |
| stereotypes | of self | of others |
| disabled | I am | I am not |
| situation | comfortable | uncomfortable |
| feelings about self | ugly, inferior, thick, stupid | |
| situation | hospital | home |
| previous fixator | yes | no |

**Context:**
in situations where others treat participants as different (actual vs. perceived)

**Strategies for managing:**
covering up
avoiding
rejecting

**Intervening conditions:**
past experience
knowing others
sensitivity to the experience of others

**Consequences:**
reduced sense of deviance

**Figure 4.4** The core category.

themselves were still at a fairly simplistic level and did not appear to reflect the content of the categories any longer. Theoretical codes, as identified by Wilson and Hutchinson (1996), were then developed and applied. The considerations made in revising the labels is presented below.

**Becoming aware:**
This was originally labelled 'shock'; however, this label was seen as too static and did not reflect the process that patients seemed to work through. This was therefore relabelled 'becoming aware'. Further consideration given to this category made the researcher feel that becoming aware also implies some form of passivity. In fact, what clients appeared to be doing is more actively going out to work out the implications of the presence of the frame. The label 'synthesizing' seemed to reflect more the process that they passed through.

**Getting over it:**
This seemed to be about the need to get over a low-level physical period during which the need to *be* well overrode the need to *look* well. Again, the label was considered to be too passive. Most people get over periods of illness, and some people try harder than others. Again, the individuals in this study seemed to work towards the goal of physical wellness. To imply more directedness in their activities the category was relabelled 'energizing'.

**Avoiding stares, avoiding questions, hiding it** and **stepping out:**
Originally, these were four separate categories and related to the notion that people were objectified by others. This was then related to the notion of deviance. However, further consideration of the data showed that each of these categories had two parts. First of all, there was the notion that they were aware that people applied stereotypes to both appearance and disability. At first there seemed to be passivity in the awareness that this was occurring to themselves. This notion was labelled 'passive receiving' and seemed to be about their perception of these stereotypes. However, an active reaction to these stereotypes, as applied by others, was their response. This was labelled 'restoration of self'. This represents the reactivity in their responses as purposeful in reducing the sense of deviance they experience as a result of the perceived and actual application of stereotypes by others.

# Process development

As Morse (1994) points out, grounded theory should be process-orientated, allowing for changes over time and identifying stages and phases that individuals go through. Using the process model (Strauss and Corbin 1990), the author began to look at how systematically the data so far could be applied to a process. The diagram in Figure 4.5 represents how the model appeared. Note that the model has concepts that are related to each other and are time and context bound. At this stage, the reader can now compare this to the preliminary conceptual framework to see how the ideas have moved on.

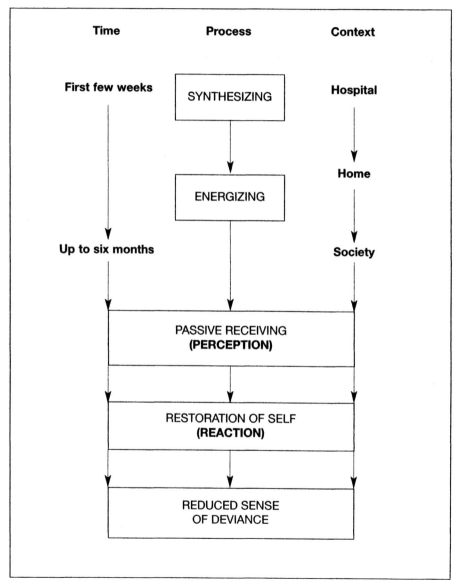

**Figure 4.5** Model of adjustment.

## Explicating the storyline

The researcher had, by now, developed a sense of how the story would appear. He therefore took the advice of Strauss and Corbin (1990) and began to write the essence of what had been discovered through many hours of data analysis. The story seems to be about seven very different individuals who had undergone limb-reconstruction procedures for a variety of reasons. In essence, they tend to be treated as deviant by a public willing to apply stereotypes because of their appearance and apparent disability.

Initial feelings regarding the presence of the fixator seem to be emotional rather than physical and relate to their perception of the appearance of the fixator. In the hospital environment, there seems to be no sense of deviance experienced. During this early phase, they tend to be **synthesizing** their feelings towards the fixator and coming to terms with its presence. Their sense of deviance is not experienced to a great extent at this point, because there are others around them in a similar condition. Also at this early stage and once the clients are in their own home environment the emphasis seems to be about regaining physical strength (**energizing**), which takes priority over their appearance.

However, once the participants appeared in public, there is a very different experience. The clients enter **passive receiving mode**. This is where they become aware of the actual or perceived **actions** of onlookers towards their appearance. They become aware that they appear different and are treated differently – society tending to treat the physically disabled as mentally disabled as well. In addition, they feel as though people stare at them and there is a tendency to be questioned about the limb, which makes participants feel as though others miss the person inside.

As a result of the **actions** of the onlookers the participants **react** in ways by which they attempt to reduce the sense of deviance they experience and thus make some attempt to **restore the self**. People often react adversely to the appearance of the limb. For some participants, particularly those with past experience, this is not a great issue. However, for others it has a negative effect on their self-image. They feel it necessary to cover their limb using a variety of techniques in order to prevent onlookers seeing it.

Because of their appearance, participants may be subject to a staring and questioning public, which again affects their self-image. Past experience also helps individuals cope with this, but for others it may lead to a reduction/change in social activity to prevent themselves becoming an object of curiosity.

The clients are often required to use a wheelchair and register as disabled. These symbols of disability are seen as creating a negative image as a result of the actual/perceived responses of others; consequently, they begin to refuse to use these symbols associated with stereotypical views. Participants felt comfortable in situations where there were others sensitive to their needs/experience.

## The literature

The literature was used in a number of ways throughout this study. This has been undertaken in line with the work of Chenitz and Swanson (1986).

- The literature was first reviewed in order to justify the need for the study.
- It was then utilized during theoretical sampling to assist the researcher to develop and refine the emergent concepts.
- The final stage was to compare it with the developed theory in order to be able to recognize and identify its differences and similarities.

Hutchinson and Webb (1991) specifically identify the difference of the final phase from the others. In the writing-up phase, the literature is integrated into the findings, and occasionally findings are compatible (or contradictory) with existing theories. They feel that presenting this correspondence is essential to a good study. To justify this action further the author also refers to the notion of the generalizability of the study. Eisenhardt (1989) feels that, overall, tying the emergent theory to the existing literature actually enhances its generalizability, particularly as the findings often rest upon a limited number of cases. In doing this, the researcher takes the findings of the study and examines them in the nature of other contexts, therefore allowing some degree of generalizability (Morse 1999).

For each of the concepts identified within the theory, and the theory as a whole, literature was considered in terms of its differences and similarities.

## Assessment of credibility

Miles and Huberman (1994) feel that part of the assessment of the credibility of the research is to identify whether negative cases and alternative explanations have been considered. In reality, the author had given consideration to other cases that may have provided alternative avenues for inquiry, and also cases that could have provided contrary evidence to the findings. The following is a discussion of the processes undertaken when considering the possibility of alternative explanations and negative cases.

## Alternative explanations

Patton (1980) points out that once the evaluator/analyst has described patterns, linkages and accompanying explanations that have emerged from the analysis it is important to look for rival or competing themes or explanations. As he suggests, the search for alternatives was done both inductively and logically. First of all, the researcher looked at organizing the data in such a way that they might lead to different findings; secondly, the researcher examined the data for instances that might support hunches. During both these processes, the author was not seeking to disprove alternatives but to look for data that provided the best fit.

The first alternative explanation focused on the concept of the physical aspects of the process. Here were a group of previously able-bodied individuals who had elected to undergo surgical treatment to correct some physical anomaly that resulted in either functional and/or aesthetic problems. As a result of the treatment, they had become physically dependent (see below) to varying degrees, an example of a category that was developed during the early part of analysis.

**Being dependent:**
**Participant 2:** The hardest thing was I was the sort of person that couldn't sit down for ten minutes, always up and about. I can't just jump up and do things, I have to wait. That's the hardest thing. I just miss being able to get up and go out in the car. That's all it is with me, I just miss my physical well-being.

In a sense the author felt initially that the disability might have some bearing upon the sense of physical self and their subsequent dependence. To pursue this line of investigation further would have possibly uncovered data relating to such; however, in order to overcome this problem, the researcher referred to the notion of best fit. Patton (1980) feels this is when the researcher considers the weight of the evidence for best fit between the data and the analysis. In this instance, while the researcher admits that there is evidence to suggest that this is a relevant phenomenon, there was insufficient evidence in early and subsequent interviews to suggest that it is relevant when compared with the amount of data related to the other categories identified as pertinent to the study.

The second alternative explanation that was given some consideration in the early stages was the idea of the effect of the treatment on the sexuality of the client. Obviously, the frame had substantial presence in the persona of the individual and affected the way clients acted, dressed and appeared. An example of a very early category is as follows.

**Dressing differently**
**Participant 1**: I quite enjoy wearing skirts. It's more feminine. It's the only way to cover up the frame.

Participant three also felt that his masculinity was affected as a result of his experience. He was previously an outgoing young man who was 'left alone' as a result of his appearance and activities, then:

**Participant 3**: As soon as I had this accident, lost all this weight, and ... my partner's pushing me around. I mean, I was like an old man. I was very frail. Like she said we went out together and we got broke into . easy pickings sort of.

The notion of the concept of sexuality having some bearing on the process was also given consideration in view of Patton's notion of best fit. Again, while the researcher saw this as relevant to the developing theory, the idea that it may be a core category was refuted early on. Using Miles and Huberman's (1994) 'wait and see what happens' policy, the researcher found that the participants did not highlight sexuality as a problem in their own expression of their experience. Therefore, the category was not used as a rival explanation but to complement the categories of **passive receiving** and **restoring the self** as clients perceived and reacted to the stereotypes applied to them.

**Negative case analysis**

Patton (1980) feels that negative case analysis is closely related to the testing of alternative explanations. He feels that considering instances and cases that do not fit increases the understanding of patterns and trends. Judd et al. (1991) further feel that it is not standardization that makes qualitative research systematic but negative case analysis. In practice, the researcher had a great deal of concern with the selection of a negative case. To identify one he felt meant potentially making and listening to value judgements. To ask the clinic staff for someone who might not fit in with the greater picture of things could result in the identification of a 'problem patient', that is one that did not fit into their picture of what the 'ideal' patient should be. Obviously, this would be selected through a completely different theoretical lens from that of the study.

However, one patient in particular interested the researcher, being identified as a potential participant by the limb-reconstruction nurse specialist.

When the participant was given an overview of the intentions of the study and some of the findings to date, he said it was perhaps no use interviewing him, as he did not have any of the experiences and problems identified by others. In saying this, he had identified himself as a potentially good negative case for analysis. The researcher informed him that the important issue in this study was to look at the variety of experiences which people were having, after which he agreed to participate. The following data extracts demonstrate how the evidence collected from this particular participant started to make the researcher question the findings at this point in the study.

**Synthesizing:**
When asked about his initial perceptions of the frame the participant replied:
**Participant 6:** There was no problem really. I'd had a video of it before; so I knew what it would be, basically what it would be like.

Also when asked about the people seeing his frame in the first few days he replied:
**Participant 6:** I'd had pins before in a previous hospital . . . so . . . mainly the visitors that came to see me were those that had already seen the video.

The researcher here refers back to the category perceiving stereotypes of appearance and asks the reader to note that response of the participant. In this case he saw no problem in people looking at his limb. Nor did he mind the onlookers seeing the frame. In fact, he saw no reason why the frame should be covered to prevent others from seeing it.

**Participant 6:** I'd wear shorts or anything; so ... I don't bother covering it up.

Reading through the transcript of this particular participant's interview made me start to question the credibility of the theory. It seemed that this particular client's experience did not fit well with that of the others interviewed so far. It seemed that he was coping fairly well with the limitations of the frame and the effect it had on his self-concept. Yet, the author didn't fully understand why this must be so. This meant a return to the transcript and a more thorough reading and further analysis. After undertaking this exercise, the researcher began to realize that a frequently occurring statement/notion was the fact that he had previous experience of a fixator and seemed well adapted to the fact that people would stare and asked questions. In fact, this was identified in the theory as an 'intervening condition'; it seemed from this interview, and one other client who had previous experience of the process, that they had already gone through an adaptive process and were able to come to terms with their present situation much easier.

On reflection, the author is also unsure as to whether or not this constitutes a negative case. In reality, all the data did fit under the categorical labels identified. What it did do was add depth to the properties and dimensions of these as identified. However, what it did not appear to do was provide a true exception. On reflection, this may actually be more representative of the 'extreme case' (Miles and Huberman 1994); nevertheless, they identify this as equally important for analysis if the theory is to have depth and credibility.

**Member checks**

Streubert and Carpenter (1995) also identify that another way of confirming the credibility of the findings is to perform member checks. They identify that the purpose of this exercise is to have those people who have lived the described experiences validate that the reported findings represent their experiences. In order to do this, the researcher met with the individuals on an informal basis at the outpatient department. All participants agreed that in some way they could see their experiences being represented by what was being discussed, and the researcher then felt comfortable in reporting the findings to the wider health care community. To some extent this was more constructive than having another colleague check the analysis as this often led to conflict in approaches and perspectives. The participant has to be the greatest assessor of credibility.

# Conclusion

Grounded theory is a very complex qualitative methodology involving many phases of data collection and analysis that occur simultaneously over extensive periods of time. However, the methodology proved very useful in eliciting the experiences of a group of adult individuals undergoing limb-reconstruction procedures.

It is important to develop a good interview technique as rich and in-depth data need to be collected. Constant comparison of the materials collected is important in developing the concepts that are relevant and need to be integrated into a logical and orderly theory that describes a process over time. An in-depth knowledge of the literature and its relevance to the theory is essential. In essence, it is a time-consuming, though rewarding, methodology.

# References

Benton DC (1996) Grounded theory. In Cormack DSF (ed.) The Research Process in Nursing (third edition). London: Blackwell Science.

Blumer H (1969) Symbolic Interaction: perspective and method. Englewood Cliffs, NJ: Prentice Hall Publishing Co.

Burns N, Grove SK (1987) The Practice of Nursing Research: conduct, critique and utilisation. Philadelphia, Pa: WB Saunders.

Chenitz CW, Swanson JM (1986) Qualitative research using grounded theory. In Chenitz CW, Swanson JM (eds.) From Practice to Grounded Theory: qualitative research in nursing. Menlo Park, Ca: Addison-Wesley

Cicourel AV (1973) The Social Organisation of Juvenile Justice. New York: Wiley.

Clarke L (1992) Qualitative research: meaning and language. Journal of Advanced Nursing 17(2): 243-252.

Cormack DFS (1984) The Research Process in Nursing. Oxford: Blackwell.

Cormack DFS, Benton DC (1996) Data presentation. In Cormack DFS (ed.) The Research Process in Nursing (third edition). Oxford: Blackwell Science.

DePoy E, Gitlin LN (1993) Introduction to Research: multiple strategies for health and human sciences. St. Louis, Mo: Mosby.

Eisenhardt KM (1989) Building theories from case study research. In Pandit NR (ed.) (1996) The creation of theory: a recent application of the grounded theory method. The Qualitative Report 2(4): 1-14.

Glaser B (1978) Theoretical Sensitivity. Mill Valley, Ca: Sociological Press.

Glaser B, Strauss AL (1967) The Discovery of Grounded Theory: strategies for qualitative research. New York: Aldine.

Goffman I (1963) Stigma: notes of the management of spoiled identity. New Jersey: Prentice Hall.

Grbich C (1999) Qualitative Research in Health: an introduction. London: Sage.

Holloway I, Wheeler S (1996) Qualitative Research for Nurses. London: Blackwell.

Hutchinson SA (1986) Grounded theory: the method. In Munhall PL, Oiler C (eds.) Nursing Research: a qualitative perspective. Connecticut: Appleton Century Crofts.

Hutchinson SA, Webb RB (1991) Teaching qualitative research: perennial problems and possible solutions. In Morse JA (ed.) Qualitative Nursing Research: a contemporary dialogue. London: Sage.

Judd CM, Smith ER, Kidder LH (1991) Research Methods in Social Relations (sixth edition). New York: Harcourt Brace Jovanovich.

Kuzel AJ (1992) Sampling in qualitative inquiry. In Crabtree BF, Miller WL (eds.) Qualitative Research Utilisation. Newbury Park, Ca: Sage.

Marshall C, Rossman GB (1995) Designing Qualitative Research (second edition). London: Sage.

May KA (1991) Interviewing techniques in qualitative nursing research: concerns and challenges. In Morse J (ed.) Qualitative Nursing Research: a contemporary dialogue. London: Sage.

Mead GH (1934) Mind, Self and Society. Chicago, Ill: University of Chicago Press.

Miles MB, Huberman AM (1994) An Expanded Sourcebook: qualitative data analysis. London: Sage.

Morse JM (1994) Qualitative Health Research. London: Sage.

Morse JM (1999) Assessing and Applying Qualitative Research. International Institute for Qualitative Methodology. Post-conference workshop held at the University of Alberta, Canada, 19 June 1999.

Morse JM, Field PA (1996) Nursing Research: the application of qualitative approaches (second edition). London: Chapman and Hall.

Patton MQ (1980) Qualitative Evaluation Methods. London: Sage.

Polit DF, Hungler BP (1995) Nursing Research: principles and methods. Philadelphia, Pa: Lippincott.

Porter S (1996) Qualitative research. In Cormack DFS (ed.) The Research Process in Nursing. London: Blackwell.

Sandelowski M (1986) The problems of rigour in qualitative research. Advances in Nursing Science 8(3): 27-37.

Schutz A (1962) Collected Papers I: the problems of social reality. Martinus Nijhoff, The Hague, 64. Collected Papers II: Studies in social theory. Martinus Nijhoff, The Hague, 67. The phenomenology of the social world. Lehart F (trans.). In Leiter K (1980) A Primer in Ethnomethodology. Oxford: Oxford University Press.

Silverman D (1993) Interpreting Qualitative Data: methods for analysing talk, text and interaction. London: Sage.

Stern P (1993) Eroding grounded theory. In Morse J (ed.) Critical Issues in Qualitative Research Methodology. Thousand Oaks, Ca: Sage.

Stern PN, Holloway G, Penson I (1982) The nurse as a grounded theorist: history, processes and uses. Review Journal of Philosophy and Social Sciences 7(6): 200-215.

Stratton P (1996) Systematic interviewing and attributional analysis applied to international broadcasting. In Howarth J (ed.) Psychological Research: innovative methods and strategies. London: Routledge.

Strauss A (1987) Qualitative Analysis for Social Scientists. New York: Cambridge University Press.

Strauss A, Corbin C (1990) Basics of Qualitative Research: grounded theory procedures and techniques. Newbury Park, Thousand Oaks, California: Sage.

Streubert HJ, Carpenter R (1995) Qualitative Research In Nursing: advancing the humanistic perspective. Philadelphia, Pa: Lippincott.

Swanson JM (1986) The formal qualitative interview for grounded theory. In Chenitz WC, Swanson JM (eds.) From Practice to Grounded Theory. Menlo Park, Ca: Addison-Wesley.

Weiner CL, Wysmans WM (1990) Grounded Theory in Medical Research. Amsterdam: Swets and Zeitlinger.

Wilson HS, Hutchinson SA (1996) Methodologic mistakes in grounded theory. Nursing Research 45(2): 122-124.

# CHAPTER FIVE

# Illuminative case studies

LORRAINE ELLIS

## Introduction

The study (Ellis 2001) this chapter comprises arose out of a long-standing personal and professional interest in Continuing Professional Education (CPE), further fuelled while I was a novice researcher involved in a funded research project. As a lecturer in nursing, I was afforded the opportunity to work on a project funded by the then English National Board (ENB): An Evaluation of Pre- and Post-registration Education to Promote Autonomy and Independence of Older People (Davies et al. 1997). One phase of the project centred on evaluating the effects of a number of ENB 941 courses ($n = 6$) using a quasi-experimental pre- and post-test design. Originally, it was intended to use a randomized controlled trial (RCT) design, but methodological and practical constraints such as the lack of a standard intervention (that is ENB 941) and difficulties in generating a sufficient sample size meant adopting a quasi-experimental approach instead (Ellis et al. 2000). The failure of the proposed RCT caused me to reflect on the appropriateness of an experimental approach to evaluating CPE, more recently referred to as Continuing Professional Development (CPD). In familiarizing myself with the methodological underpinning of the experiment, I became increasingly aware of the tensions between the central tenets of positivism and the multifaceted nature of most CPD. Central to the experimental method is control, randomization and manipulation, concepts I found difficult to square with the complexities of learning in diverse environments. I began to question how the experimental method could take account of, or seek to control, such complexity. This questioning led me to search for an alternative approach that might provide a more complete and comprehensive account.

As a neophyte researcher, I was drawn to the body of literature on interpretive methods concerned with the study of social phenomena in their natural settings. Such methods seemed to hold promise for the study of CPD as they paid greater attention to the processes and broader context within which CPD operates. Compared with the experiment, they offered a differing set of lenses through which to view the world. In respect of the present study, as will be discussed more fully as the chapter unfolds, both pragmatic and intellectual considerations pointed towards using a case study approach realized within a modified illuminative evaluation. This chapter therefore provides an account of a journey of discovery and learning that led to a PhD.

This chapter is organized under a number of headings that reflect the stages of the research process and unfolds chronologically. Stages of the research process include the literature review, research strategy and methods and the findings. Each section opens with a series of questions and issues that arose as the study proceeded.

# The literature review

- What is the purpose of the review?
- What is the best way to undertake the review: searching and organizing the literature?
- What are the key findings of the review and what is the best way to present them?
- What are the emerging research questions?

### Purpose of the review

The role of a literature review and the influence of existing knowledge more generally is a highly contested and widely debated topic within qualitative research. While some contend that the literature should not be consulted prior to data collection and analysis for fear of bias (Glaser and Strauss 1967), several writers present a case for getting to know everything there is about the setting, the culture and the study topic prior to entering the field in order to avoid 'reinventing the wheel' (Morse 1994, Guba and Lincoln 1994). As I had already been involved in the delivery of CPD for several years and had recently been a participant in a major research study, it seemed naive to assume that I would enter the field without prior knowledge. It was therefore considered important that this knowledge was as comprehensive as possible both for me to be able to recognize any potential for bias and also to locate the study relative to the existing body of knowledge. The intention was not to identify and follow *a priori* themes or hypotheses but rather, as Morse (1994) asserts, to recognize leads without being led. Put differently, my aim in consulting the literature was to become a wise and smart researcher but not a directed researcher.

## Searching the literature – the process

Searching the literature involved a systematic process using a variety of techniques to ensure a comprehensive and, wherever possible, complete identification of the body of literature on CPD in nursing. The literature search covered the 50-year period from 1945 to the beginning of 1996. An update of the literature from 1996 to 2001 (study completed) was presented as part of the discussion and conclusion. The review process involved reading the classic and the lesser-known texts, the theoretical as well as the empirical literature, and published and unpublished works. A comprehensive list of relevant sources was developed through a combination of computer and manual searches. The databases that were used to identify and locate the literature on CPD were CINAHL (Cumulative Index of Nursing and Allied Health Literature), ENB (English National Board for Nursing, Midwifery and Health Visiting Health Care), INI (International Nursing Index), ERIC (Educational Resources Information Centre), RCN Nurse ROM and Dissertation Abstracts International (DAI). The keywords used to search the literature included continuing professional education, post-registration nurse education, continuing education, nurse education, benefits of continuing education, higher education and education and training. Electronic searching was complemented with a hand search using an incremental approach that allowed for the cross-checking of sources. Meta analyses of studies evaluating the effectiveness of CPD were also used.

## Organizing the literature

There is a diverse range of literature on CPD that presented a challenge as how best to distil this information in a coherent and meaningful way. To aid this process a thematic approach was adopted with the potential relationships within and across the themes being summarized diagrammatically. These themes emerged through a process of sifting and organizing the literature systematically as though analysing a set of data. In so doing the review process provided a detailed account of those aspects of CPD that were relatively well rehearsed, while also identifying apparent tensions and areas that received limited attention.

## Findings of the literature review

Four broadly related themes emerged, each consisting of a number of sub-themes: the policy and legislative context of CPD, the benefits of continuing education, barriers that inhibit the uptake of CPD and barriers to subsequent change to practice following CPD. Together these themes capture important characteristics of CPD, highlighting those factors potentially contributing to an effective system. A full and detailed account of the literature review is reported elsewhere (Ellis 2001).

As noted at the start of this chapter, my initial interest in the evaluation of CPD arose out of a long-standing professional involvement, further fuelled by my involvement in an ENB-funded study. This was originally designed as an RCT and later changed to a quasi-experimental method. Even then, however, limitations were apparent, and I was left with the feeling that experimental methods generally are too deterministic to capture adequately the complex environment in which CPD operates. Such perceptions were reinforced following the review of the literature that revealed deficits in a number of areas, particularly in the consideration of the context of CPE, the need to reflect differing view points and in charting the impact, whether positive or negative, over time. Two sets of perspectives emerged as being of particular interest, those of practitioners nominated for courses and their managers.

## What are the emerging research questions?

At this stage in the research process a number of broad research questions or issues were identified including:

• What are the perceptions, expectations and experiences of nominees and managers pre-programme?
• How do these factors influence the way that nominees experience the programme?
• What is the nature of the educational experience itself and how does this affect their perceptions?
• What do nominees and their managers see as the outcomes of the course immediately following the programme?
• Do these perceived outcomes change over time?
• What factors influence perceptions of programme outcomes over time?
• What factors influence whether practitioners are able to stimulate change following the programme?

In addition to the above, I also felt it important that the views of educators be obtained and that their perceptions of the programme as written (in the curriculum), and delivered (in the classroom), be compared with those of nominees and their managers.

With the above research questions in mind, a search of the methodological literature was undertaken in order to identify an appropriate research design. This next section contains a brief consideration of the paradigms for evaluating CPD, providing an explanation and justification for the approach that was adopted.

# Research strategy and methods: choosing the right approach

- What strategies are available to study CPD?
- Which strategy is best suited to answer the research questions?
- Which strategy is best suited in this context?
- The possible contenders: case study and illuminative evaluation
- Illuminative case study: an emerging design

This next section provides an account of the overall strategy and methods used to evaluate a short focused programme, the ENB 941 (Nursing Older People). The background and context of the study are outlined together with a consideration of evaluation paradigms providing the rationale for the research strategy that formed the basis of this PhD study. Subsequently, attention is turned to the more specific methods that were adopted.

My interest in CPD and my involvement in a funded research project served to highlight the limitations of the classical experimental approach to the evaluation of educational programmes, and initiated a search for more holistic and context-focused methodologies. The original study had been designed as an RCT but the methodological and practical constraints resulted in a change to a quasi-experimental design. Several of the methodological constraints and limitations of traditional experimental evaluation raised by this funded research feature in the literature (Ellis et al. 2000). It is perhaps worth noting, however, that these issues are especially pronounced when the study involves human subjects in an educational context where the researcher is dealing with the complexities of learning and attempting to measure its effects in an equally complex clinical environment (Ellis 1996).

Few studies evaluating CPD fully acknowledge the complex multidimensional nature and processes of continuing education but instead follow the outcome-focused tradition of positivism. Interest tends to centre on the product of nurse education, on whether the curriculum works and if the behavioural objectives have been met not on how the curriculum is interpreted, applied and received. Guba and Lincoln (1994) assert that traditional models of evaluation suffer from similar deficits, namely that they:

- fail to acknowledge the fact that different groups may not value the same outcomes or objectives, therefore definitions of success will vary
- rely too much on a positivist view of the world based on an objective and value-free reality
- strip programmes of their context and therefore fail to provide important explanations as to how and why programmes work or not

It was just such concerns that provided the impetus for the present study. In seeking an alternative approach, it would have been comforting to be able to write that decisions had been driven primarily or exclusively by methodological concerns, that I was free to select whichever approach provided the most cogent set of philosophical arguments. However, few researchers are afforded such luxury, and decisions are influenced by practical, as much as by theoretical, issues with the exigencies of life often being the determining factor. In the present instance, I was already engaged in a study and was committed to finishing it. It therefore seemed prudent that, as far as possible, and without compromising my desire for an alternative approach, the study build upon existing work. Moreover, upon completion of the study, I was required to return to work as a full-time educator with there being little prospect of pursuing a project full-time. Registering for a part-time PhD would allow me a day a week for research (or the equivalent in blocks of time), with the possibility of more time being available when teaching loads were lighter. Any study would therefore need to be broadly achievable within such parameters. Given my existing familiarity with the ENB 941 and the interest this had generated, common sense dictated that a study which sought to evaluate this programme was the best approach to follow.

In some respects, therefore, this major methodological decision, while not quite a *fait accompli*, nevertheless afforded an opportunity not to be passed over lightly. A review of the interpretive approaches suggested that a case study design, focusing on one of the ENB courses may be appropriate.

### Case study: a brief consideration

Case study has many proponents within educational research (Parlett and Hamilton 1987, Stake 1995), but until recently it has tended to be viewed as the poor relation of educational evaluation. Yin (1994) argues that there is a need for a new interpretation of case study that raises its status from that of a weak sibling to a method of first choice. Similar arguments were made a decade earlier when, during the early 1960s, the case study was still viewed with caution by many, lacking the credibility of more established experimental approaches.

While this reticence was in large measure due to the traditional dominance of experimental methods, there was also a relative lack of clarity as to what a case study constituted. In seeking greater consensus, authors agreed that case study was not a method *per se* but rather a family or palette of methods (Stake 1995), with case study being neither intrinsically qualitative or quantitative. Indeed, Stake (1995) suggests that case study is not a methodological choice at all but rather a choice as to what to study, that is, it focuses on a particular instance or case. The research case study differs from its use in teaching, medical or legal situations, but case studies are nevertheless characterized by their concentration on particular instances or, as will be highlighted below, occasionally on a small number of particular instances. On this basis my decision to study the ENB 941 strongly suggested the wisdom of using a case study approach.

In his most recent (at the time the study commenced) publications on case study, Stake (1995) suggest that there are three broad types of case study that can be adopted. He does not see these as being hard-and-fast variants that compartmentalize a study but rather as fluid with there inevitably being some overlap in any given study. He describes these three types as:

- intrinsic case study
- instrumental case study
- collective case study

In an *intrinsic case study*, the researcher is primarily interested in the case itself, not what it might say about similar cases but because the case is intrinsically interesting. There is no intention or desire to generalize beyond the single case considered. In contrast an *instrumental case study*, although still the study of a single instance, is interested primarily in what that instance might say about a wider class of related instances. Stake (1995) contends that in such a situation it is the phenomenon or issue(s) that drives the study rather than the case itself. The ability to make some inferences beyond the single case is therefore important. This is not viewed as generalization in the statistical sense but rather the desire for a modified (and presumably enhanced) understanding by providing new insights. A *collective case study* is a variant on the instrumental model which involves the use of multiple related cases to enhance the degree of generalization possible.

For the present study my interests lay not in the ENB 941 *per se* but rather what a study of the ENB 941 might have to say about CPE more generally. This clearly suggested the use of an instrumental case study with the issues identified at the end of the last chapter providing the main focus. However, as the study unfolded and the informants were followed to their clinical environments, the project moved towards a collective case study, with informants' perspectives serving to provide insights into a range of practice issues.

The case study seemed to provide a good way forward, allowing me to pursue my interest in qualitatively orientated approaches to evaluation. However, this decision still left other important considerations open. As Stake (1995) points out, the case study is not a choice of method but of what to study. Therefore, it was necessary to select a particular approach from the palette of methods available. This led to a search for a methodological approach within which to explore the case study.

# Illuminative evaluation – a way forward?

In my reading of the case study literature, the work of Parlett and Hamilton (1987) on illuminative evaluation surfaced a number of times. Stake (1995) makes explicit reference to Parlett and Hamilton, particularly their notion of a 'progressive focus'. Indeed, Stake's own suggestion, that as a study unfolds it moves from very generic questions to more clearly focused issues, was clearly heavily influenced by the idea of a progressive focus. Although I was vaguely familiar with the term 'illuminative evaluation', I was less clear as to exactly what it meant, and this prompted a detailed reading of Parlett and Hamilton's (1987) original description. What follows is a brief account of the central elements of illuminative evaluation.

Illuminative evaluation was developed in response to the perceived limitations of traditional evaluation (Parlett and Hamilton 1987) and emphasized interpretation rather than measurement and prediction. Unlike traditional evaluation models illuminative research is designed to take account of the wider context in which educational programmes function. Accordingly, illuminative research stands firmly and unambiguously within the alternative socio-anthropological or naturalistic paradigm (Parlett and Hamilton 1987) that is primarily inductive in nature. Illuminative evaluation was developed for general mainstream education and focuses on two main areas, the instructional system and the learning milieu.

## The instructional system

The instructional system, or curriculum intention, is a central component of illuminative evaluation and concerns the formal and 'idealized specification' of the programme (Parlett and Hamilton 1987). However, Parlett and Hamilton assert that the curriculum undergoes modification in the process of being implemented in a complex and naturally existing context. Elements of the curriculum are, according to Parlett and Hamilton (1987):

> emphasised or de-emphasised, expanded or truncated, as teachers, administrators and students interpret and reinterpret the instructional system for their particular setting.

Thus, the programme objectives may be reordered, redefined, abandoned or forgotten. The notion that the curriculum is transformed through the process of interpretation further compromises the assumptions of traditional evaluations, where the curriculum is used as a blueprint against which the outcomes of the programme are measured. Indeed, research that takes the programme in its original form as a self-contained and independent system is problematic, for in practice it manifestly is not. Parlett and Hamilton (1987), mindful of curriculum modifications through interpretation, suggest the need to catalogue details of the programme, including the programme's aims and objectives, its pedagogic assumptions and teaching styles, the course content and overall philosophy. Features of the educational effort that appear to have had desirable results are important in helping to explain events and outcomes. Notably, illuminative evaluation focuses on the study of 'innovatory programmes', the evaluation forming an integral part of the innovation to aid decision-making. Of an even greater importance, however, is the context in which the curriculum unfolds. This is termed the 'learning milieu'.

## The learning milieu

The learning milieu comprises the sociopsychological and material environment in which students and teachers work together. Essentially, this milieu represents a complex network of cultural, social, institutional and psychological influences acting within the *classroom* context. Unlike traditional evaluation, an illuminative model attempts to take account of these variables considering the interplay of numerous factors, including:

- organizational imperatives and constraints such as administrative and financial considerations
- teaching methods, subjects and the assessment of students
- individual teacher characteristics, such as professional orientation, experience and private goals
- student perspectives and preoccupations

Following a detailed consideration of the instructional system and the learning milieu, an illuminative evaluation does not produce neat and tidy results, nor is it explicitly intended to isolate causal inferences. Rather, as Parlett and Hamilton (1987) assert, its purpose is to illuminate issues such as what is it like to be participating and what are the scheme's significant features, recurring concomitants and critical processes? In addressing such issues, the intention is to aid understanding in a number of ways by:

- shaping discussion
- disentangling complexities
- isolating significant influences
- raising the level and focus of debate

Parlett and Hamilton (1987) point out that illuminative evaluation is a generic approach rather than a method, and that within any given study it is up to the researcher to document and justify the particular methods adopted. Nevertheless, as with the advocates of case study research (Stake 1995), they suggest that the primary methods will be a combination of observation, interview and documentary analysis. Moreover, in using an illuminative evaluation, they promote the idea of a progressive focus (moving from broad general issues to more tightly circumscribed but not prescriptive questions) following an iterative sequence comprising:

- getting a general feel for and becoming knowledgeable about the scheme or programme under study
- selecting a number of phenomena, groups or opinions for more detailed study
- trying to establish some general principles or 'recurring concomitants' that might help to provide potential explanations

The conceptual similarities between the above sequence and Stake's (1995) contention that the qualitative case study moves from a 'foreshadowed' problem (a broad, generic area of concern) to the identification of more specific issues to the formulation of potential assertions (or loose hypotheses) are readily apparent and further reinforced the complementary nature of what I termed an 'illuminative case study'.

In their original, and now seminal, account, Parlett and Hamilton (1987) are at pains to point out that their description of illuminative evaluation is not a prescription or a blueprint but rather a broad set of principles to be adopted by the individual researcher according to particular circumstances. In the present context, while I was convinced of the importance of the instructional system and the learning milieu, it seemed that the potentially most significant influence on the effectiveness of CPD was omitted, that is the impact of the clinical environment into which the practitioner returns. The literature clearly highlighted the importance of the receptivity or otherwise of the practice arena, and in a longitudinal study, such as the one proposed, a consideration of this seemed absolutely essential. To account for this, therefore, an additional major component was added to Parlett and Hamilton's original conceptualization and this was termed the 'practice milieu'. As will become readily apparent in the findings presented in the following sections, the influence of the practice milieu was central to an understanding of the experience and impact of CPD.

## Activating an illuminative case study

- How best to go about an illuminative case study?
- What forms of information or data are congruent with the chosen research strategy?
- What sources of information or data are accessible within the study's timeframe?

Having made important decisions about the use of an illuminative case study, it was necessary to decide how best (and most realistically) to collect the data required. The texts on both case study (Stake 1995) and illuminative evaluation (Parlett and Hamilton 1987) suggest three main approaches: observation, interviews and documentary analysis. For the present study, observation – while desirable – was not feasible. The limited time available to the researcher, the labour-intensive nature of the observation and the need to consider the practice milieu of several participants effectively precluded observation. The emphasis was therefore placed on documentary analysis and interviews. The major focus of the documentary analysis was the course curriculum and supporting documents for the ENB 941, while interview data were collected from the educators delivering the ENB 941, the nominees to it and their managers.

## Sampling and negotiating access

- Why this population and sample size?
- Generating the sample – some of the difficulties
- What information will potential participants require in order to consider participating in the study?

Sample selection has a considerable effect on the research process, with qualitative researchers in particular being criticized for failing to describe their sampling strategy in sufficient detail. Lack of detail makes interpretation of the findings difficult and affects the replication of the study. As noted earlier, owing to a series of pragmatic considerations, the sampling strategy adopted in this research was convenience or opportunistic sampling, with the informants being identified through my membership of the ENB-funded project. In the process of generating a sample for the funded project, I was able to identify those practitioners nominated to a forthcoming ENB 941 offered by the school of nursing in which I worked. Nominees and their managers were made aware that I was a nurse educator employed by the school of nursing but that I had no involvement with the ENB 941. Educators were already aware that I was an employee of the school. My background was considered a distinct advantage as I shared a common culture with all the participants and therefore was more likely to gain 'backstage' data and less likely to be misled.

However, despite having access to information on those nominated to the ENB 941 and a knowledge of the system of contracting, generating the sample was not without difficulty for several reasons. While the school held a list of the names of the forthcoming ENB 941 nominees and their place of work, the list proved to be incomplete and was out of date. Some of the potential research participants, when contacted, indicated that they had withdrawn their application or were unaware that they had been nominated. Identifying the nominating manager also proved problematic as some nominees were unclear as to who had nominated them to the ENB 941. Difficulties identifying the sample were exacerbated by the short timeframe. The list of ENB 941 applicants was available just three weeks before the ENB 941 commenced, leaving little time to fully brief and interview the research participants. Educators to the programme were understandably less difficult to identify since I had knowledge of those associated with the ENB 941. The difficulties encountered in generating the sample reflected issues about the selection process that emerged as part of the data analysis.

Notwithstanding these difficulties, a sample was identified, with each nominee and respective manager being invited to participate in the study and consent to being interviewed before the nominee commenced the ENB 941. Initial contact with the participants was made over the telephone, and their potential involvement in the study was detailed as follows:

- the study aimed to evaluate the nominee's ENB 941 and from a variety of perspectives, including nominees, managers and the course leader
- participation involved being interviewed at six-monthly intervals pre-course, immediately post-course, and at six and 12 months post-course
- interviews would normally be tape recorded
- each interview would last approximately 30 to 60 minutes
- total confidentiality was guaranteed

# Ethical considerations

- What ethical principles guided the research?
- How were these principles applied in this context?
- What features of the research design and methodology served to protect the interests of the participants?

Ethical considerations form an important and fundamental aspect of research involving human beings as care must be taken to avoid doing any harm. Each of us, whether designing and carrying out research or acting as a critical consumer of research findings, has a responsibility to develop a knowledge and understanding of ethical issues. Much has been written on research ethics, and numerous guidelines for conducting research are available. Such guidelines were developed and formulated following grave concern over the research carried out on inmates of the concentration camps during World War II as exposed during the Nuremberg Trials.

In designing and conducting this longitudinal study, I made a conscious effort to adhere to ethically sound principles to ensure that the research was acceptable to the research participants. In so doing, I attempted to adhere to four ethical principles concerning the protection of participants: beneficence, non-maleficence, respect for autonomy and justice.

Beneficence holds that we should try to do good. It could be argued that the intention of research to add to knowledge is implicitly beneficial. In the context of this longitudinal study this of course was more likely to be gauged in the longer term. Closely linked to beneficence is the second principle of non-maleficence, in other words that if one cannot do good one can certainly try to avoid doing harm. Protection from harm may be enhanced where the researcher concerns themselves with issues of informed consent and the right to privacy. The principle of non-maleficence was especially pertinent in the context of this research as I was both a researcher and educator working in the same institution that offered the ENB 941. Interviewees gave of their time and energy and allowed access to their private thoughts and experiences in the course of this study. I also had unlimited access to the curriculum documentation that was owned principally by those educators who delivered the programme. In these terms, the research participants may incur costs.

In the context of this study, therefore, adherence to the principle of non-maleficence is about ensuring issues of anonymity and confidentiality and that participants are made aware of the research findings and possible implications for their practice and also that, if the occasion arises, they have the opportunity to withdraw from the study at any time without detriment in any way.

One of the characteristics of personhood is the ability to make free choices about oneself and one's life – to be self-governing. The principle of autonomy is said to be at the heart of informed consent and was an important consideration in this study. Acting in accordance with the principles of respect for autonomy the researcher is required to ensure that participants give free and informed consent. Informed consent means that those who participate in research give their consent while in possession of all the relevant information necessary for them to make a proper choice. A closely linked concept is confidentiality, and this concerns the rights of individuals to control information about themselves. Here it is necessary that the researcher ensures that the participants are not only offered anonymity and confidentiality but also protected throughout the study and subsequently. Free and informed consent is, according to some writers, difficult if not impossible to obtain as there will always be an imbalance of power and knowledge between researcher and participants. For example, the participants may be unfamiliar with the methodological intricacies of a particular design of study. This longitudinal study meant interviewing the participants on several occasions thereby increasing their familiarity with the study and possibly countering the imbalance of power in this context. The way in which consent was obtained and anonymity ensured is described briefly below.

Despite informed consent being the right of every individual, it is difficult to know when one can claim that it has genuinely been given and achieved. In the present study, potential participants were given information about the project and written, informed consent was obtained. Information about the longitudinal study included the purpose of the study, my role in the study and the nature of their commitment, including the number, frequency and approximate length of the interviews. This was an important consideration since their involvement would extend beyond the funded project. Potential participants may be unwilling or unable to commit to this level of participation due to work obligations. Prolonged participation in this study increased the amount of time spent away from the practice setting. In acknowledgement of this, consent to participate in this study was sought at the outset and reaffirmed throughout, thereby providing informants with the opportunity to withdraw from the study at any point. To support participants in their decision, they were also informed that withdrawing from the study would not jeopardize their nomination to the ENB 941 or create prejudice as a colleague. Consent was also obtained to tape record the interviews, and participants were made aware that on completion of the study the tapes and transcripts would be destroyed or returned to the informants. Accordingly, a conscious and concerted attempt was made to keep the participants fully informed from the outset and on an ongoing basis throughout this longitudinal case study recognizing my responsibilities to the informants.

Justice as a principle of research ethics is about fairness and that research participants are treated alike when the situation demands. The type of research undertaken is explicitly about ensuring that the knowledge gained empowers individuals to action.

Participants' privacy was protected in various ways. Data were collected, stored and reported in a manner that ensured that, wherever possible, no one but the individual concerned was aware of their source. Participants' identities were protected by assigning a code to the transcripts.

## Integrity of the researcher

Ethical approval was obtained from the Local Research Ethics Committee. However, the protection of the research participants goes beyond seeking ethical approval and is about the integrity of the researcher in carrying out the study. It was important to possess the relevant knowledge and skills to carry out this study and, as a novice researcher, to recognize the limitations of research competence. This is a minimum requirement to safeguard the well-being of research participants and to maintain professional credibility. I was also able to confirm the appropriateness of the arrangements for data management, storage, retrieval and ownership to protect participants' confidentiality and avoid introducing bias into the data sets. Prolonged contact in the field of study aided the integrity of this study providing the opportunity to develop and hone my research skills throughout the research. It is also important that the researcher recognizes and makes known any relevant conflict of interests that may influence the investigation. In the present context, I was not only a researcher but a nurse and educator, and therefore when seeking consent to participant in this study all the informants were made aware of this, and this was reiterated throughout the series of interviews. Participants were also made aware that, while I had no involvement with the ENB 941 programme, I was an employee of the school of nursing and therefore there was the potential for a conflict of interest.

The researcher must also be satisfied that the knowledge that is being sought is not already available so that they are not wasting the time of the research participants and resources. Prior to the study, a review of the literature was undertaken and omissions in the body of knowledge indicated. Having described how ethical considerations were addressed, attention is now turned to the interviews themselves.

## Interviews with nominees and managers

- What factors influenced the number and frequency of interviews?
- How much notice were interviewees given prior to each interview and why?
- Where were the interviews conducted and why?
- What were the benefits of repeated interviews over time?
- What factors influenced changes in the sample size over time?

Nominees to the ENB 941 and their service managers were interviewed four times over an 18-month period, once before the course commenced, immediately post-course and at six and 12 months post-course. Repeated and regular contact with the same sample was integral to the project design and its attempts to capture both unique and typical patterns of development that had usually gone unexplored in previous studies. In all but one instance the participants were interviewed separately, with each interview being face to face. The exception was during one interview where the nominee and manager were interviewed together due to time constraints.

All the interviews were by prior arrangement with at least one week's notice so that the interview would not interfere with the participants' practice. Most practitioners requested that they be interviewed in the afternoon, as there were additional staff on duty at this time. Recognizing the additional demands that an interview may have placed on the informants, most interviews lasted between 45 and 60 minutes, and generally this proved sufficient. The exceptions were in instances where the respondent clearly wished the interview to continue further.

For the most part the interviews were held at the participant's place of work and during work time. The exceptions were three nominees who were interviewed in their own home because they were either no longer practising or had moved to another setting. Informants were usually interviewed in a quiet room that was some distance from the main practice area and free of a telephone. These measures went some way to help safeguard against interruptions and other distractions. Interestingly, the further into the study the fewer the interruptions and the more at ease the participants became. While a matter for conjecture, this was possibly because the informants had become familiar with the routine of the interview and were therefore likely to anticipate and take measures to prevent interruptions. Similarly, repeated contact meant that the informants were more at ease with the interviewer.

Although the intention had been to keep the same sample throughout the study, some variation proved inevitable due to changes in the working arrangements of informants. In order to give an indication of how the interviews progressed over the course of the study, this information is summarized in Table 5.1.

**Table 5.1** Changes in sample size over the stages of the study*

| Participants | Pre-ENB 941 | Immediately post-ENB 941 | 6 months | 12 months | Total no. of interviews |
|---|---|---|---|---|---|
| Nominee | 15 | 13 | 12 | 11 | 51+1* |
| Manager | 21 | 15 | 17 | 15 | 69 |
| Total sample size over the study | 36 | 28 | 29 | 26 | 121 |

\* one of the nominees withdrew from the ENB 941 one week into the course and was therefore interviewed
  at this point also, making the total number of nominee interviews 52

# Interviews with educators

Educators to the ENB 941 were also interviewed in order to complement the curriculum analysis and to gain a more complete picture of the ENB 941. Educators were interviewed separately and face to face. Their contribution to the nominees' ENB 941 varied from acting as the course leader to being responsible for a specific module. Educators were interviewed to gain insight into their interpretation and implementation of the written curriculum. One-to-one interviews afforded the opportunity to elucidate potential differences and shared understandings. Interviews with educators were by prior arrangement with a minimum of a week's notice so as not to interfere with work commitments. These interviews were carried out in the school of nursing in a quiet room determined by the educators themselves.

# Data-analysis strategy

- How were the data analysed?
- Why were the interviews analysed following each interview?
- What process undertaken earlier in the research guided the analysis?
- Why was it important to keep a record of the process of analysis?

The curriculum and the interview data were analysed through a process of 'content analysis', a term loosely applied to a variety of approaches rather than a single conceptually distinct technique. Latent analysis was used to analyse the curriculum document, although some descriptive frequencies were included as they offered valuable insights about certain aspects. Analysing the curriculum involved reviewing passages and paragraphs to identify the major thrust or content of the section. These were then assigned to themes. Relevant data were therefore colour coded and organized under broad headings or categories, with an indication of whether they constituted either explicit or implicit outcomes noted in the margins. Regularities and recurring issues were identified through this process, with searches made for patterns and connections within and between identified categories. Where there were shared meanings, categories were combined. These themes and their meanings were subsequently cross-checked and referenced with respect to both the perspectives of the educators and also the experiences of the nominees.

All of the interviews were tape recorded, transcribed verbatim and analysed following each interview. These early results were then used to inform subsequent interviews. There were 121 interviews with nominees and their managers, producing extensive volumes of data on which it was necessary to impose some conceptual order. Analysis was guided, but not directed, by the issues identified in the literature review, the purpose being to highlight any potential areas of interest. However, consistent with the canons of case study, the main goal was to provide an account that captured as fully as possible the informants' meanings. Familiarity with the data is a crucial first step in qualitative research and was achieved through detailed readings and by the process of constant comparison aided by latent content analysis (Glaser and Strauss 1967).

The following description provides an account of the data analysis in order to give a sense of how this process was applied in the context of a longitudinal study. The analysis involved a detailed reading and re-reading of the transcripts so that I became very familiar with the data. This continued throughout the 18 months of data collection with responses being visited and revisited, looping backwards and forwards looking both for similarities and unique aspects. Immersion in the data in this way meant that gaps in my understanding were highlighted in order that they could be explored further in subsequent interviews. Therefore, each interview was informed by the analysis of data previously collected. The responses of each nominee and respective manager were also analysed comparatively, then located with respect to the responses of other nominees and their managers across the entire sample. This process of analysis helped to retain each individual's story or account over time. This was necessary for comprehension but also facilitated the merging of accounts essential for synthesis and theorizing.

In terms of the more mechanical process of data analysis, several writers offer practical guidance on how to handle data. In the present study, initial categories and codes were identified following the first detailed reading of individual transcripts in order to gain a sense for any emerging themes before the focus shifted to a line-by-line analysis. Data were highlighted and preliminary categories and codes freely generated in an attempt to take account of all the data. Paragraphs, sentences or even individual words were assigned a category, a process that was repeated throughout the series of interviews. Revisiting the data was essential to a full understanding of both the individual and collective story, particularly as the volume of data increased as the study progressed. As analysis continued, indices of saturation were sought, such as repetition of themes, until no new data were emerging at a given point. Categories and their potential associations were mapped onto a large sheet of paper together with the emerging themes, as these were confirmed or refuted through the process of constant comparison. Mapping was especially useful for considering the data at each stage of the study and across the study as a whole. It provided the main mechanism whereby synthesis and theorizing were achieved.

Keeping a record of this process was an integral part of the analysis and helped retain familiarity, so that during interviews it was possible to mentally locate participants' responses in the context of their previous data. At the end of each interview, I also recorded any new themes or insights that appeared to be emerging and any contextual information that might be useful in the subsequent analysis.

## Issues of quality in qualitative research

Despite the robust process of analysis, confidence in the resultant findings and therefore their contribution to the body of knowledge ultimately rests upon the trustworthiness of the data and the research process. Several authors have criticized qualitative research for failing to clearly address issues of validity and reliability. Presenting a credible account enhances confidence in the findings and means that it is imperative to report upon issues such as validity and reliability if the research is to be seen as meaningful. However, this is no simple matter, as the whole issue of what 'counts' as appropriate criteria is a vexed one. An essential first step is to recognize the different concepts and terminology used in addressing issues of quality/ trustworthiness in qualitative work.

Writers in the field of naturalistic inquiry draw parallels between the concepts of validity and reliability as used in quantitative research and their qualitative equivalents. One of the earliest and most widely cited attempts to address the issue of rigour in naturalistic inquiry was made by Lincoln and Guba (1985), who in their now seminal text outlined a model for considering the integrity of qualitative research. A full and detailed account and application of this model in the context of this research can be found in Ellis (2001).

## Summary of findings

This next section presents a summary of the curriculum as written and interpreted by educators followed by the interviews with students and their managers.

- What were the central findings of the content analysis of the curriculum?
- How did these findings differ from the interviews with educators?
- What is the best way to present these data?

### The curriculum as written

Analysis of the curriculum revealed a number of emergent themes: the aim and purpose of the ENB 941, the structure and management of the course, the content taught and teaching methods, assessment and evaluation. A synthesis of these findings indicated that the curriculum consisted of an intentional message together with a series of underlying assumptions.

For example, on the one hand the overall aim of the programme is to improve the care of older people, yet the document tended to stress the development of generic knowledge and skills. Emphasis was also placed on the application of theory to practice, although rarely in connection with the care of older people despite this being the stated aim of the programme. Similarly, while the title of each module referred to the older person, the indicative content tended to be generic in its orientation. Neither did the curriculum explicitly state that the 'older person' is to be the focus for the development of the students' written work. While the curriculum identified the clinical environment as a barrier to change, there was no mention of how the student might overcome such barriers.

### The curriculum as interpreted – educators' views

The findings of the interviews with educators ($n$ = 3) reflected the tensions and contradictions revealed in the curriculum analysis. For example, consistent with the findings of the curriculum analysis, research and reflection were said to be important features of the ENB 941, although educators were unclear about how these aspects related to the stated aim of the programme. The educators also questioned the inclusion of a range of topics that were taught on the ENB 941 and considered these to be unrelated to the care of older people, for example topics such as study skills and sociology.

These views concurred with the analysis of the curriculum where generic knowledge and skills were emphasized over the care of older people. Educators also stated that the course assessment aimed to promote developments in the nominees' practice. Nonetheless, they also indicated that the students often chose topics for their portfolio entries that bore no relevance to the care of older people. Moreover, these inconsistencies appear to mirror the contradictions that were evident in the curriculum between the document's stated aim to improve the care of older people and its generic emphasis and the evaluation of the ENB 941 being centred on the nominees' experience of the course. The tendency of the informants to evaluate the educational processes over outcomes may have been reinforced due to the educators being responsible for only one module. Evaluation that is process-orientated without reference to the outcomes of the whole programme is likely to produce an incomplete picture of the educational experience.

In summary, therefore, the analysis of the curriculum for the ENB 941, together with the views of educators, provided information about the stated intentions of the curriculum and its underlying assumptions, while also revealing a number of contradictions. Educators' interpretation and perspectives on the course also served to highlight the congruence between the curriculum and educators' perceptions and interpretation of the ENB 941. Together these findings provided some insight into how the programme was likely to be received and experienced by the nominees.

The next section presents a brief summary of the findings of the interviews with nominees and managers presented longitudinally: pre-course, immediately post-ENB 941 and six and 12 months post-course respectively. First, attention is given to how I arrived at the decision to present these data chronologically.

## Interviews with students and their managers

The decision about how best to present the respondent's story was a vexed one: there were so many data on which to report. Thus, I experimented and rehearsed different approaches until eventually settling for one that seemed to do full justice to the respondent's story reporting the participant's story as it unfolded chronologically. In distilling the essence of the results, it proved helpful to think of these in a number of broad areas relating sequentially to each stage of the longitudinal study in terms of those factors influencing the nominees and managers at various points in time, namely:

'Going in'                    – factors pre-course
'Coming out'                  – immediate post-course perceptions
'Reaping the benefits'        – perceptions at six months post-course
'Carrying it on'              – perceptions at 12 months post-course

Nominees' accounts were presented first as this reflected the sequence in which most of the interviews took place and therefore helped to contextualize these data and locate them contemporaneously as they emerged.

### Going in: pre-course perceptions

'Going in' presented the nominees' and managers' perceptions and expectations before the ENB 941 commenced. If the processes described by the nominees and their managers are compared with those promoted within the literature as part of this study, it became apparent that almost none of the criteria suggested are met. Rather than the planned and systematic approach that is advocated, the experience of the nominees paints a picture of an *ad hoc* and arbitrary system of selection, often based on chance. This relates to both nominees and their managers.

Few of the nominees voiced any real desire to attend the ENB 941 *per se*, rather it was a matter of 'taking what's going'. Even those nominees who could give explicit reasons for their attendance rarely related these directly to working with older people; it was simply their intention to 'keep ahead of the game'. These apart, other motivations related to getting time out from a hectic work environment in order to 'recharge their batteries'. Despite the lack of clear aspirations, all nominees accepted their place

enthusiastically yet had concerns mainly relating to the academic component ('Can I hack it?') and the difficulties of balancing competing demands
('juggling too many balls'). Few had engaged in discussion with their managers, and so it was a case of 'second guessing' their expectations.

Conversely, managers often provided quite different, and sometimes
contradictory and inconsistent, accounts. Responsibility for the selection
of candidates varied, although all the managers said they were clear on
their selection criteria. Paradoxically, however, often none of the criteria
were applied to the ENB 941 candidates. Even where there were some
explicit expectations and a purposeful and planned process was adopted,
decisions were still usually based on generic criteria rather than those specific to the care of older people. Generally, there was no assessment of
candidates' needs and no discussion about their respective expectations.
Thus, the extent of pre-course planning and support for nominees in making the right educational choice was severely limited in most instances.

Ironically, the reasons candidates asked for CPD were often those that
their managers considered inappropriate. For example, time out was seen
as a legitimate reason by most nominees, while their managers thought
otherwise. There was also evidence of, largely unintended, bias and dis-
crimination, particularly relating to nominees with family responsibilities,
those working on nights and/or occupying junior positions.

Despite the random selection process, most managers had expectations
of the nominees post-course, although these were not communicated to
the nominee ($n$ = 16). Managers also had very limited knowledge of the
current ENB 941 despite many of them having completed the course
previously. They were largely unaware of nominees' concerns, especially
relating to the academic components of the course.

*Coming out: perceptions immediately post-course*

'Coming out' presented the views of the nominees and their managers
immediately post-course. These data provided useful insight into nominees' experience of the curriculum and importantly the receptivity of the
practice milieu post-course. The support nominees received from managers varied with some being aware of the nominees' experiences and
outcomes while others had very limited or no knowledge. Nonetheless,
even when managers were aware of nominees' plans for change, support
was rarely planned. For the most part, managers remained unaware of the
quality of the nominees' educational experience, tending instead to report
how they themselves had benefited from CPD.

Interestingly, these interviews highlight the potentially negative effects
of CPD for managers and nominees alike, findings not previously reported
in the literature. For nominees, these difficulties related to their personal
circumstances, while for managers the tension between supporting CPD

and maintaining practice was problematic. Nominees also perceived the practice environment to be compromised, demonstrating levels of insight that the managers rarely displayed with respect to nominees' personal circumstances. These differing perspectives highlight the lack of discussion and planned follow-up, creating frustration in some nominees who were keen to share the benefits they had gained. Indeed, while motivation was considered an important factor, a supportive practice milieu figured prominently as a potential barrier to improvements in care.

### Reaping the benefits: perceptions six months post-course

This chapter has presented nominees' and managers' accounts of the effects of the ENB 941 six months post-course, providing further insights into its outcomes and the receptivity of the practice milieu. Managerial support remained limited and unplanned, with most managers displaying scant knowledge of the benefits of the nominees' course. This was reflected in their tendency to speak in general terms about themselves rather than focusing on the nominee. The ENB 941 continued to positively affect four of the six nominees, who identified benefits immediately post-course. These practitioners all worked in areas where the practice milieu was more receptive and initiatives were encouraged. Consistent with the literature, the benefits of CPD appear more likely to be realized in a climate that encourages and facilitates autonomy. While the range of benefits often went unnoticed by managers, some noted benefits that were not mentioned by the nominees, such as an interest in furthering their education. These findings highlight the value of interviewing both managers and nominees. Consistent with the nominees' accounts, managers also observed a more individualized approach to care, although this was the only benefit on which both parties were agreed. Interestingly, it was not until six months post-course that managers noticed a more positive attitude towards the older person, whereas nominees indicated that their attitudes had altered immediately post-course.

The importance of a receptive practice milieu was now mentioned by both managers and the nominees, who interestingly emphasized differing aspects. Understandably perhaps, managers highlighted organizational change, while nominees centred on the lack of managerial support and limited resources. Managers also reflected the difficulties of introducing technology as part of care in a climate where the traditional view of nurses at the bedside prevailed. Interestingly, those managers who were more circumspect about the benefits of the ENB 941 also tended to emphasize the deficits of the curriculum. Nominees' enthusiasm for change was difficult to sustain, particularly where the practice milieu was less receptive. Certainly, motivation appeared to be a key factor in whether the benefits of CPE were fully realized, as noted in the literature.

Both groups of informants again reported the negative outcomes of the ENB 941 and CPD. CPD was thought to raise aspirations causing nominees to seek work in other areas and diminish resources further, or to create disappointment and frustration if change was not realized. While a matter of conjecture, staff may have been denied continuing education to prevent them from seeking opportunities elsewhere. Another significant finding is that education had, for some, made their role less rewarding, with their efforts to introduce change creating tensions and distress. Understandably, owing to the negative effects of their experiences, these practitioners were now disillusioned.

What is of interest here is that the data obtained immediately post-course and that six months later varied to some extent, with both nominees and managers reporting differing emphases. This highlights the potential value of ongoing evaluation. However, once again, there was little evidence of a systematic structure to evaluation in any of the practice settings. Even in supportive environments, well planned and rigorous procedures for appraisal were not in evidence, with most of the canons of good practice identified in the literature review being conspicuous by their absence.

*Carrying it on: perceptions 12 months post-course*

Nominees continued to benefit from the ENB 941, though fewer mentioned the benefits at this interview than previously. However, one participant described benefiting from the course for the first time. This suggests that reflection plays an important role in realizing the benefits of CPD for some participants. Positive outcomes continued to be evident including holistic assessment and challenging stereotypes, as well as a further interest in education and increased confidence and maturity. This was particularly the case amongst more mature nominees who had previously doubted their academic abilities.

The practice milieu as a barrier to change continued to feature and was more prevalent than at any other time post-course. The emphasis now firmly centred on the lack of managerial support, their random nomination and the managers' inability to advise on the suitability of the ENB 941. Paradoxically, even when nominees were managers themselves, they remained indifferent to the support needs of other ENB 941 candidates, possibly suggesting a cycle of indifference.

# Conclusions

This chapter has presented an account of a journey of discovery and learning that led to a PhD. In relaying this journey, every attempt has been made to retrace the research steps with accuracy to produce a detailed and, wherever possible, unsanitized account. The background to the development of this study clearly suggests that a multitude of factors influenced the choice of design and methodology – personal, practical and philosophical. These factors had a bearing on the available choices and the decision-making process, and are measures of the multiple and often competing demands in which real-world research is often conducted for, while undertaken as part of a formal programme of study and scholarly driven and resolute, this research did not occur within an academic vacuum divorced from the complex reality of practice. Indeed, as has been illustrated, the converse was true.

Integral to the PhD thesis was a reflexive account of the research process (Ellis 2001). This reflexive account not only served in recounting the story of events here but, of significance, was instrumental in maintaining the integrity of the research. Science would have us believe that reality may be subject to control, as in the RCT (Ellis et al. 2000). Real-world research, and particularly qualitative research, is inherently messy, which requires creativity and imagination on the part of the researcher, particularly in upholding the integrity or validity of their research. Illuminative case-study research represents such an attempt.

# References

Davies S, Ellis LB, Laker S (1997) Evaluation of Pre- and Post-registration Preparation for the Care of Older People. Report for the English National Board (ENB) for Nursing Midwifery and Health Visiting. London: ENB.

Ellis LB (1996) Evaluating the effects of continuing professional nurse education: researching for impact. Nursing Times Research 1(4): 296-306.

Ellis LB (2001) Continuing professional education for nurses: an illuminative case study. University of Sheffield: Faculty of Medicine (PhD thesis).

Ellis LB, Davies S, Laker S (2000) Attempting to set up a randomised controlled trial. Nursing Standard 4(21): 32-36.

Glaser BG, Strauss AL (1967) The Discovery of Grounded Theory: strategies for qualitative research. Chicago, Ill: Aldine.

Guba EG, Lincoln YS (1994) Competing paradigms in qualitative research. In Denzin NL, Lincoln YS (eds.) Handbook of Qualitative Research. London: Sage.

Lincoln YS, Guba EG (1985) Naturalistic Inquiry. London: Sage.

Morse JM (1994) Emerging from the data: the cognitive processes of analysis in qualitative inquiry. In Morse JM (ed.) Critical Issues in Qualitative Research Methods. Thousand Oaks, Ca: Sage.

Parlett M, Hamilton D (1987) Evaluation as illumination: a new approach to the study of innovatory programs. In Murphy R, Torrance H, (eds.) Evaluating Education: issues and methods. London: Paul Chapman.

Stake R (1995) The Art of Case Study Research. London: Sage.

Yin RK (1994) Applications of Case Study Research. London: Sage.

# CHAPTER SIX

# Ethnography

LEE CUTLER

## Introduction

The aim of this chapter is to give the reader an introduction to ethnography. In doing so, the chapter will consider the key elements of ethnography and, through an example research study, how it can be applied in attempting to answer a research question. The chapter will also consider some of the difficulties I experienced while undertaking an ethnographic study.

Ethnography is concerned with culture and cultural knowledge. In an attempt to understand a particular culture, we must strive to understand people from a cultural perspective. It is not true that culture can only be studied from a qualitative perspective. Frequently in the media we are presented with the latest findings about what percentage of a given group in society behaves in a certain way. This is the application of statistics and a mathematical approach to the study of culture. It can give great breadth to our understanding. However, this book and this chapter are concerned with gaining a deeper understanding through qualitative research.

Qualitative study of culture requires that we understand what people do and say, how they relate to one another, what they believe, what their customs and rituals are as well as how they interpret their experiences. Attempting to gain such a deep understanding may often require that breadth of understanding be sacrificed. The beginnings of contemporary ethnography were marked by studies of far-off civilisations by western anthropologists who produced their descriptions, or 'ethnographies', of those cultures. These pioneering ethnographers had a focus to their study, and it was a focus on one cultural group that allowed such depth in their findings.

The ethnographic approach, its focus and outcomes have a great deal to offer nursing and health care. Patients and nurses are members of cultures and as such a great deal of how they think, behave and interact may be determined by culture and can be revealed and explained through ethnog-

115

raphy. Thus, ethnography is a highly useful method that has been applied to such groups in order to understand what has traditionally been very difficult to articulate – the special and often invisible art of nursing. One particular example is Savage's (1995) study of interactions between nurses and patients; however, many more exist across health care specialities and patient groups and can be found listed at the end of this chapter.

It is through applying ethnographic methods in new and challenging contexts that the approach has undergone expansion and refinement, and so it continues to evolve. This dynamic communicates the real world of research, its challenges and complexities, its paradoxes and compromises. Some of these will be addressed in this chapter.

## Overview of my focused ethnographic case study

As part of my postgraduate studies, I was required to undertake a research study. I chose to investigate the cultural context in which learning from critical care education programmes might be applied. I hoped that this might help to inform the educational programme content of such courses. Below is an overview of the study and its background.

Recent literature considering critical care in the NHS has acknowledged that the critically ill are not just to be found within the walls of intensive care units (ICUs) but in increasing numbers across acute clinical areas, such as the medical and surgical ward. Clearly, the increasing severity of illness in the acute-ward area demands a great deal of the nursing staff in these busy areas. *Comprehensive Critical Care* (DoH 2000), which is the nearest thing critical care has to a national service framework, laid down many mandates in relation to the changing face of critical care. Amongst these were educational mandates for nursing staff in acute-ward areas, namely that they should receive training to deal with the increasing numbers of critically ill in their care. My study took place in the context of these and many other changes in nursing, health care, critical care and nurse education.

Within the literature, there is an unequivocal assertion that continuing professional education should, ideally, influence practice and improve patient care. However, the relationship between education and practice, or theory and practice, is an energetically debated one. The theory-practice gap, as it has come to be known, carries with it the ideas that just because theory exists this does not mean that practitioners know about it, understand it, that it is applicable and helpful to practitioners or that it is refined and informed by the changing practice of nursing.

It was my contention at the beginning of the study, and, for some time previously, that developing and facilitating successful educational experiences for practitioners requires that the educationalist understands the context in which the practitioner will go forward and try to apply what they have learned. Building on the work of Rogers and Shoemaker (1971), three main concepts have been distilled and found to be associated with successful adoption of innovation and learning in practice. The concepts can be defined as follows:

- *Compatibility* is the degree to which the programme content is compatible with the needs of the nurse and the organization.
- *Relative advantage* is the degree to which the learned material is perceived as better than that which it supersedes.
- *Practical applicability* is the extent to which learned material can be applied, trialled and experimented with in the real-life practice of nursing.

Without understanding the real-life experience of working in the culture of acute-ward care, I would argue that it is difficult, if not impossible, to design new educational innovations that meet the perceived learning needs of acute-care nurses and, more specifically, to offer content that is compatible and offers relative advantage and practical applicability.

These concepts were used to form a tentative framework that guided the formulation and conduct of the study (see Figure 6.1). These three concepts were used within this study to inform a series of informal, open-ended interviews that probed the real-life experiences of nurses caring for critically ill patients in one acute surgical ward chosen as a case-study area. It was hoped that the study could reveal part of the culture of ward-based critical care nursing and use this information to expand our understanding of how education needs to fit with such culture and practice.

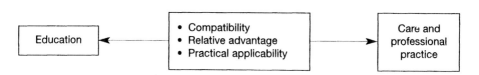

**Figure 6.1** The relationship of educational content to care and professional practice: the proposed conceptual framework that guided the study

The findings informed a more sophisticated view of these three concepts and their possible relationship with nursing practice in a ward culture. They also allowed a novel view of the issues and paradoxes ward nurses faced when caring for critically ill patients. These have direct implications for the course content of educational programmes that might aim to address the knowledge and skill deficits described in recent Government reports on critical care. A more extensive discussion of the findings is included later in the chapter.

# Features of ethnographic research

Opinions about ethnography, its essential elements and what make good ethnographies, are probably as numerous as ethnographers. It is not the purpose of this section to give a full discussion of the literature pertaining to ethnography, for this the reader is directed to the references in this chapter. The aim here is to give a succinct description of what is seen to be at the core of a study that makes it an 'ethnography' or leads one to describe the approach as 'ethnographic'.

Several key themes link ethnographic studies. These include:

1. a focus on culture
2. the researcher's role in the study
3. the product of the study

## A focus on culture

Culture is about the things that individuals have in common because they share group membership. This membership does not exist in the formal sense, through a written contract for example, but comes through shared presence, knowledge, understandings, language, values and behaviour to a greater or lesser extent.

It may be quite daunting to consider entering a culture alien to our own and undertaking a formal study of it. Where does one begin? How much does one probe, describe or try to understand? In reality, nurse ethnographers rarely enter a field with a very broad remit and a blank slate wishing to undertake very holistic ethnographies. There is often a burning question or specific personal interest. The researcher may ask, 'How is stress perceived and dealt with within a team of nurses?' Nursing ethnographies also often focus on a relatively well-defined group, or a large group that can be justifiably reduced to a smaller case study for the practicalities of a research study.

## The researcher's role in the study

The researcher is the one who is curious enough to ask questions, to be interested and, in the final analysis, the one to possess the resourcefulness and tenacity to make a study happen. However, the specifics of the ethnographic researcher's role are the concern of this section. The goal of the ethnographer is to describe and understand the chosen culture. It is not uncommon in anthropology to see solitary researchers entering the chosen culture and staying there for some time. The reality for many contemporary nurse researchers is that time and resources set natural limits on the study and the researcher's stay in the culture.

During the stay, many types of data will be gathered to enhance understanding. In describing the data-gathering function of the researcher, the reference to 'researcher as instrument' is often seen in ethnographic literature. This phrase is intended to convey that the nature of the data to be collected is so enmeshed in the culture that it can only be gathered by one who has some intimacy with the group being studied and with the information shared within that group. Thus, the researcher is using individual skills and qualities to achieve the necessary proximity or acceptance within the group. Once this is achieved, the researcher becomes the conduit through which data can be channelled.

While the terms 'conduit' and 'researcher as instrument' have been used here, this does not mean that the researcher is cold, procedural and detached from the data, or that there is a lack of any analysis in the field. There is often an ongoing cyclical process of data collection and analysis. Critical thought about the data as they are gathered challenges the researcher to probe in different directions – asking previously unconsidered questions as likely means of deepening and broadening understanding. This critical thought may also involve reflection on how the data challenge the researcher's prior knowledge or assumptions about the culture. The ability of the researcher to engage in such cognitive processes is often described as 'reflexivity'. This process involves comparing the insider's ('emic') perspective with the researcher's own perspective as an outsider ('etic'). The terms 'emic' and 'etic', often used in ethnographic literature, also refer to what people are observed to do by the researcher as outsider versus what they say that they do. The 'reflexivity' that results from the dynamic between the two perspectives is thought to be synergistic and helps in the creation of a third dimension, or a new perspective.

The 'field' and 'fieldwork' are said to be some of the hallmarks of ethnography. The field is a physical setting, the boundaries of which are defined by the researcher in terms of institutions and people, as well as their associated interest. Fieldwork is a set of actual research tasks carried out in a chosen setting or location. It is the role of the researcher to decide on the nature of the field and fieldwork. Having done this, it is the researcher's job to gain access. Gaining access does not simply mean entering the building. It is the human contents of the building that the ethnographer is really interested in. In my study, for example, gaining access did not merely relate to obtaining legitimate ethical and managerial permission to undertake the study. In a very informal and tacit way, true access to the field was gained by attempting to build a rapport with the staff that might be part of the case study. This is characteristic of ethnography since the extent to which the researcher is accepted within the group may affect how individuals portray and share their knowledge, language and behaviour, for example to someone who is an outsider.

'Participant observation' is often seen as the cornerstone of fieldwork in ethnography. For nurse ethnographers undertaking research in clinical settings such participant observation may present some challenges. I had particular ethical and professional difficulties with this element, as will be discussed below. An in-depth understanding can often only be gained through asking questions of those in the culture under study. This may be done informally as part of *ad hoc* interactions or in a more formal and structured setting, such as a tape-recorded interview that allows one to probe individuals' beliefs, knowledge, assumptions and the meaning of the language and terms they use with each other. While questions may be predetermined, as one explores the culture more questions may be generated as understanding is deepened and initial assumptions are exposed as inaccurate ways of viewing the culture.

## The product of the study

The product of research using this approach is referred to as an 'ethnography'. The ethnography may be descriptive or interpretive depending on the aims of the study and what is already known about the culture. For example, a researcher may attempt to describe a culture about which very little is known. It might be acceptable to seek description before one tries to understand some of the more complex or hidden issues about a culture. However, if a relatively well-described culture is under investigation, the researcher may seek more interpretive findings that explain complex phenomena and give more depth to what is understood.

Another thing that will determine the nature of the ethnography produced is its intended audience. For example, it may be published as a book for the general population or, by contrast it may be very esoteric and written for a particular academic or professional community. The style, content, depth of description and interpretation will all need to suit the receiving audience.

It is often customary in ethnographies to gather and present data that give a pictorial, geographical or structural dimension to the findings. For example, in my study I attempted to communicate the context of care by describing the number of beds, nurses and consultants on the ward, the complexity of the case mix and the recent changes in the nursing establishment that had occurred because of long-term sickness and the retirement or promotion of staff. Although some may present photographs, a picture of a floor plan or other diagrams, I omitted these since I tried at all costs to preserve the anonymity of the ward I studied and such diagrams would have made it more identifiable.

The description and interpretation of the culture can take several forms. For example, a narrative informed by field notes may structure the text or, as in the case of my study, the data were analysed and presented as a number of themes that were salient within the culture and which related to the focus of the study. To gain an insight into the way ethnographies are written, the reader is advised to read some of the studies listed at the end of this chapter.

**Summary**

One could be forgiven for thinking that the concepts and elements presented above can be used to structure and guide a study one is planning to undertake. However, such features do not merely come from rigidly drawing up and following a plan – rather, one could argue that often they are features that emerge within an excellent ethnography. They come through genuine interest in a culture, the enthusiasm to learn about the ethnographic approach and the tenacity to carry out an investigation, often in challenging circumstances. The concepts do not link neatly to one another. It is the author's experience that, in attempting to study culture in relation to the real world of nursing practice, these key elements present major challenges, contradictions and dilemmas. These will be discussed to some extent later in the chapter.

# How I prepared for the study

The successful execution of many excursions, projects and innovations is to a great extent reliant on careful planning. This section aims to provide an explanation of the planning and conduct of the study. It includes some of the philosophical and practical considerations that are integral to any research. Such information is a vital part of any research report for the reader who wishes to understand what was done and why.

The first step in planning the study was to decide on a research question to give the study a focus. A series of aims was also developed to inform the methods and directions of the investigation.

*The research question*

What should educational programmes aimed at preparing nurses in general ward areas to care for the critically ill contain, and in what cultural context might learning be applied?

*Aims of the study*

1. To explore the real-life experiences of nurses caring for the critically ill in an acute-ward area.
2. To explore the impediments to, and support for, the **practical application** of **compatible** educational programme content in the everyday clinical context.
3. To explore the nature of nursing the critically ill in the ward environment and to identify what educational content might be **compatible** with this nursing.
4. To explore what actions were employed, or might usefully be employed, to make a positive difference in the experiences discussed (what **relative advantage** is perceived).
5. To explore the extent to which the conceptual framework proposed in Figure 6.1 can be informed, refined or reformulated following an interpretation of the findings.
6. To discuss the findings of the study in the light of recent educational mandates regarding education for critical care and broader substantive literature.

The planning and conduct of the study is schematically represented in Figure 6.2 below.

## Articulating my frame of reference

To give a fully contextual view of the methodology it is important to discuss the 'frame of reference' since it affected how the study was planned and conducted.

A frame of reference is a structure at an abstract level. It is about the logic and meaning that guides the development of a study and enables the researcher to relate the findings to existing knowledge. A major component of the frame of reference for this study is embodied in the conceptual framework (presented in Figure 6.1 above) since this was derived from existing knowledge found in the literature. The conceptual framework served to provide a description and clarification of concepts.

However, a further important component of the frame of reference is the researcher's own 'paradigm', or belief system about the world. This represents: 'How the researcher perceives a group of concepts relate together' (Ellis and Crookes 1998). This aspect of the frame of reference is important to document since it can help the reader understand the researcher's thoughts, reasoning and conclusions.

Because paradigms reflect beliefs about the world that cannot be proven true or false, they are quite contentious and often highly personal. It

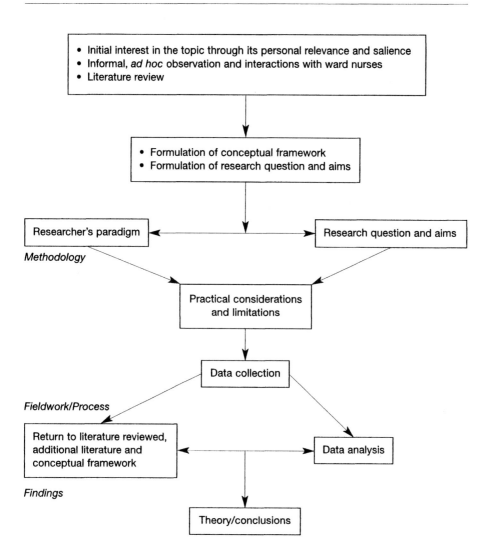

**Figure 6.2** Schematic representation of the planning and conduct of the study.

should be made clear that the beliefs expressed here are accepted as tentative and conjectural and are part of a continuing philosophical debate.

Nolan and Lundh (1998) assert that paradigms are used to propose answers to at least three sets of questions. The questions relate to beliefs about reality (ontology), knowledge (epistemology) and research methods (methodology). My view of knowledge and reality about this area of nursing was made up of several key beliefs and concerns:

- I was a lecturer-practitioner and had been charged with developing and supporting education for nursing staff caring for seriously ill ward patients. I believed that it was very important to provide education that would help nurses improve the care of these patients.
- I believed that, because I was a practitioner, my understanding of the complexities and difficulties was more up-to-date than some teachers who worked as full-time teachers in higher education.
- I believed that education had to recognize and fit with the complexities and difficulties that exist in the clinical area.
- I believed that there was much more to know about the everyday reality of this area of nursing than I knew at the beginning of the study.
- I believed that understanding the clinical context of learners' practice allowed me to develop more congruent, relevant and applicable educational programmes, and I wanted to understand more. I also wanted to help others within education, practice and possibly a wider circle develop their understanding – which I felt was lacking in some areas.
- I believed that the reality of ward-based critical care was very complex, contextual and dynamic. Such beliefs resonate with what LeCompte and Schensul (1999) have called an 'interpretive' or 'constructivist' paradigm:

> interpretivists believe that what people know and believe to be true about the world is constructed – or made up – as people interact with one another over time in specific social settings (LeCompte and Schensul 1999).

Therefore, to *truly* know about this reality (my epistemology) would be a difficult, if not impossible, goal; this was an uncomfortable realization. The implication was that, through this research, I would only be able to *construct* a view of real-life nursing. This was because the reality did not exist as a fixed external situation. To view reality as fixed, external and therefore measurable, it has been argued, is a belief from a very different paradigm – that of *positivism* (LeCompte and Schensul 1999). Unlike positivism, the findings of research influenced by constructivist, or interpretivist, beliefs are not true in a probabilistic sense. Rather, they are more or less informed and/or sophisticated. The constructs discussed in such research are not fixed but can be altered through dialogue and over time leading to new constructions or views of reality. This also helped me become more aware of the implications of my beliefs and what the results of research might lead to.

I believed that the process of seeking to increase understanding in this area of clinical practice required that I got close to the staff and study their beliefs, values and practices without attempting to control or manipulate the setting or the subjects. Such closeness would have inevitably had a bearing on the data collected, its interpretation and the findings of the study. Thus, it was acknowledged that the research process would be affected by interactions and biases between myself, as the researcher, the subjects under study and the data.

The interactions between subjects and the researcher are seen as important within a constructivist paradigm. This is because:

> the constructs or meaning systems of researchers, participants, and research partners all carry equal weight, because negotiated meaning cannot occur unless the researcher is a full participant in the process (LeCompte and Schensul 1999).

Positivists who seek to be more objective and distant from the data-controlling relationships and their effects would oppose such beliefs.

As discussed above, a feature of ethnographic research is reflexivity – or critical thinking about different perspectives of the same issue. It is not uncommon for researchers to dedicate sections of their ethnography to reflexivity. (See, for example Savage 1995.) In this way, reflexivity is perhaps made explicit. However, in my report, reflexivity was not set aside and commented on in some discrete section as though a discrete act. Rather, reflexive thoughts and my responses to them in formulating and conducting the study are to be found throughout the study integrated within the discussion. This is because I perceived that such an integrated approach allowed a more spontaneous uninhibited flow of reflexive thoughts to be documented in amongst the discussion to which they pertained.

The conceptual framework for the study (Figure 6.1), interpretation of how the components of the frameworks interact and finally my own paradigm (beliefs regarding ontology, epistemology and methodology) contributed to the frame of reference for this study. This informed the formulation, conduct and, inevitably, the findings of the study. However, the focus of this section is also to discuss the decisions made and methods used in the study. It is important for the purposes of clarity to describe how multiple factors came to influence the study methodology, and how this was put into action.

As can be seen in Figure 6.2, there was a relationship between my beliefs (paradigm) and the research question and study aims. However, this process was at a fairly abstract level and these abstractions had to be converted into a pragmatic plan for investigating the topic area chosen. What follows is an account of the decision-making process around abstract issues as well as the procedural actions of the sampling, data collection and analysis.

## Why I chose a qualitative method

The literature review revealed that there was a limited understanding of the reality of caring for the seriously ill in a ward environment and of the necessary skills and knowledge.

A decision was made that a qualitative approach was most suitable. This was because of the limited understanding, and because there was no intent to test theory, hypotheses or offer predictions, as might be the case in an experimental design. Rather, the aim was to add to the existing body of knowledge through exploration.

The term 'qualitative' has been used in many ways and can be confusing. It therefore deserves clarification here. By 'qualitative' what is meant is that the data collected were not of a mathematical or statistical type and were analysed in a nonmathematical way. There is no standard approach amongst qualitative researchers; however, they all share a commitment to naturally occurring data. Furthermore, they occupy a paradigm with similar beliefs on reality, knowledge and naturalistic methods.

> Qualitative methods are primarily concerned with in-depth study of human phenomena in order to understand their nature and the meanings they have for the individuals involved (Hunt 1991).

Within the qualitative paradigm there is great diversity and debate over methods. Some argue that researchers should stick rigidly to particular approaches, for example grounded theory or phenomenology, while others argue in favour of mixed methods, or in the evolution or adaptation of methods.

> I have no problem with researchers tinkering with a given method or inventing a new one. What I cannot abide is the author who claims to have used grounded theory but whose end product is some kind of hybrid (Stern 1994).

She continues that the whole point is 'within the parameters of science: I really don't care what you did, just tell me about it. I might learn something'.

The approach used within this study is described as qualitative, but it was not rigidly adherent to any specific methodologic doctrine. Rather, it was informed by case-study research and ethnography and as such was an eclectic qualitative approach.

Most importantly, its employment was not aimed at measuring the culture of ward critical care, manipulating the environment or subjects, or testing a hypothesis. Rather, the aim was to study the naturally existing culture in the ward and draw conclusions about what implications this had for education.

## Why ethnography?

The aim of producing holistic and contextual studies of naturally occurring phenomena is what characterizes qualitative research. However, the desired end product is what determines the type of qualitative method used. One of the goals of ethnography is to make that which is implicit within a culture explicit (Streubert 1995).

Such descriptions of ethnography as a method to study culture drew me to this approach. The idea of making visible what is hidden was appealing, and the way in which an ethnographic approach is said to enable this made good sense after I had grappled with thoughts of how best to understand a foreign culture with all its secrets.

It was my conclusion that the assumptions, or cultural unawareness, of those working outside ward areas may lead to erroneous conclusions about the capabilities necessary or lacking in ward nurses. Furthermore, simply asking ward nurses about necessary or lacking knowledge, skills or attitudes may not be fruitful, since they may not be aware of what they do not know. Put differently, they may be unaware of different ways of working since they are immersed in one culture with its own ideology, traditions, values and beliefs. However, to attempt to educate these individuals without some understanding of the culture within which they work and from which they will interpret the messages of the educator, one may argue, is at best folly and at worst arrogant. This is perhaps further complicated by the way I, as a researcher and practitioner, was immersed in different cultures from those I intended to study.

The terms 'emic' and 'etic' are common terms in ethnographic literature and they are related to the 'reflexive' nature of this approach. The emic perspective is the insider's, or informant's, view of reality. This view of what is happening and why is important in understanding and accurately describing situations and behaviours. The etic view is the outsider's framework, the researcher's abstractions or the scientific explanation of reality. The combination of these two views side by side produce a 'third dimension' (Boyle 1994) rounding out the ethnographic picture. The two disparate systems of knowledge mean that the ethnographic researcher has not to take data at face value but instead consider them as a set of inferences in which hypothetical patterns can be identified to provide theoretical explanations.

## Not just ethnography but an eclectic approach

Up to this point, the position taken and methodological decisions discussed have mainly centred on philosophical assumptions and abstract concepts. However, putting such assumptions into a pragmatic plan for action required consideration of what was possible within the time and field available.

It was neither possible nor desirable to produce an ethnography of a large number of acute wards. Furthermore, a study of the entire culture of a ward would exceed the aims of the research since the aims were centred on nurses only and, in particular, the care of critically ill individuals. From the conduct of such small-scale focused studies, various terms have emerged to describe the kind of study undertaken. Thorne (1991) suggests that nurse ethnographers rarely conduct whole ethnographies. Leininger (1985) uses the term 'mini ethnography' to describe a narrow area of enquiry. Morse (1991) argues that the term 'focused ethnographies' be used to describe topic-orientated, small-group ethnographies. Examples of such studies include Germain's (1979) *The Cancer Unit* and more recently Savage's (1995) *Nursing Intimacy*.

Boyle (1994) relates that these 'particularistic' ethnographies focus on a social unit or processes within a small group. They generally identify and help us to understand the cultural rules, norms and values and how they are related to health and illness behaviour. The term 'focused ethnography' has been used to describe this study, denoting that it had a specific focus within the study of a culture.

The term 'case study' has also been used within the literature to describe ethnographies. A case study is conducted in natural settings and is an in-depth study of the singular. Such a study of focus and of the singular, in terms of a small social group, may be criticized for failing to generate the kinds of findings that contribute to evidence-based teaching. However, Bassey (1999) cites Hargreaves (1996) when the former makes several points in defence of educational case-study research.

First of all, the notion of evidence-based teaching may be simplistic. Hargreaves, in a lecture to the Teacher Training Agency, talked of 'evidence-based teaching'. This, basically, translated into a very reductionist and simplistic view of teaching and learning. He called for research which:

> demonstrates conclusively that if teachers change their practice from x to y then there will be a significant and enduring improvement in teaching and learning (Hargreaves 1996).

Bassey's response to this statement is that teaching situations are so varied and complex that such statements can never be made with certainty. Furthermore, that to say 'do x instead of y and your students *may* learn more' is no minor change. However, we first need to understand the complexities that prevent generalizations of certainty about teaching and learning. Case-study research is advocated as one way to conduct an in-depth study of complex natural phenomena. The findings of such studies may feed professional discourse on these issues and may lead to theoretical assertions and what Bassey (1999) has called 'fuzzy generalisations'. This phrase acknowledges that exceptions to these generalizations must be recognized. Understanding human complexity is paramount.

Pictured below (Figure 6.3) is a representation of the eclectic approach utilized in this study.

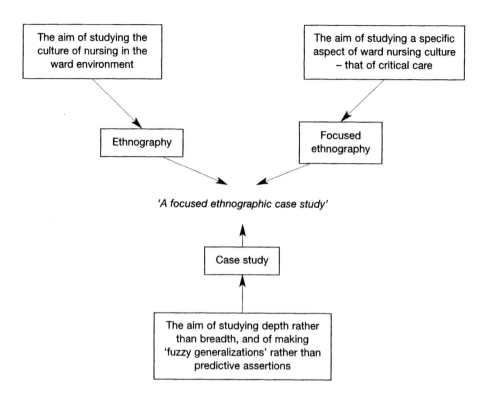

**Figure 6.3** The eclectic methodology employed in the study.

## How I approached the ethical considerations

In general, health care research is viewed as an overall good (Mathews and Venables 1998). However, there have been numerous studies in which unethical conduct by the researchers has been discovered (Burns and Grove 1993). When considering the ethical issues related to a study, it is useful for researchers to employ some kind of framework. It is not my intention here to discuss all the issues I considered; however, the framework I used is worthy of presentation together with a practical example of how its principles were carried through into the conduct of the study.

MacLeod Clark and Hockey (1989) suggest that the ethical considerations of nursing research can be clustered under five headings:

• aims and purpose of the research
• unnecessary risks or inconveniences to patients or staff
• respect for confidentiality and anonymity
• competence of the researcher
• intended use of the research findings

My major concern was to protect and reassure those who agreed to participate in the study. The way I ensured informed consent was by using a standard form with each participant interviewed. This is presented in Figure 6.4.

Further ethical challenges emerged during the fieldwork, which are discussed below.

---

*Research consent form*

**Who is conducting the study and why?**
My name is Lee Cutler. I am currently undertaking a masters degree in education at the University of Sheffield. I am required to write a dissertation based on research I have conducted around the subject of education.

**What is the study about?**
The study aims to explore the real-life experiences of nurses working in acute-ward settings. It is hoped that this will lead to an understanding of what facts and items of knowledge and skill might be beneficial for students if included in future critical-care education programmes aimed at ward nurses.

**What will happen if you agree to be involved?**
If you agree to be involved in the study, I would like to interview you about your experiences of caring for critically ill patients in an acute-care-ward area. The interview may last up to an hour and, with your consent, would be tape-recorded for future analysis.

---

**I have read the above information about the study and:**

- I agree to be involved.
- I understand that my participation is entirely voluntary.
- I consent to being interviewed (tape-recorded).
- I understand that I may withdraw from the study at any time without providing a reason or without fear of bias in any way because of withdrawal.
- I agree to give consent for data from my interview to be used in the research report and any subsequent publications that may come as a result of it, provided that the data are anonymous.
- I am entitled to privacy and that I may refuse to answer any questions I am asked without prejudice.
- I understand that the information disclosed in interview will be strictly confidential.
- I understand that the tape-recordings of the interview will be kept in a locked cupboard and that only the researcher will hear them or read the transcripts.
- I understand that the tape will be erased at the conclusion of the study.
- I understand that if, for any reason, I feel that the conduct of the research is becoming detrimental to anyone involved, I can contact those who have given the researcher permission to conduct the study

Signed:_____        Signed:_____
Lee Cutler                               (participant)

---

**Figure 6.4** Consent form used in my study.

# Some challenges faced during the fieldwork

Many challenges face the researcher while planning, conducting and reporting a study. In this section, I have attempted to share just a few of the challenges I faced while conducting my ethnography. These challenges were selected because they were particularly relevant to this methodology and to those undertaking research as non-expert practitioner-researchers.

After planning the study and gaining permission to access the field, I began my initial data collection. I had planned to observe the care of seriously ill patients and then interview the nurses involved at the next opportunity. Participant observation is seen by many as the cornerstone of fieldwork in ethnography and has been employed in nursing ethnographies of acute and critical care previously (see, for example, Savage 1995 and Seymour 2001). It is central to identifying and building relationships important for the future of the research. It is also an opportunity to attend and witness events that outsiders would not be invited to attend and as a way of seeing what people actually do.

I had come to believe that doing ethnographic research meant that it was imperative to make participant observation a major part of my data collection. However, attempting to turn this ideal into a reality was a learning experience that highlighted an ethical dilemma.

I had contemplated the issues that I may face in my role as an observer of nursing. I was concerned that I might be drawn into helping with care or even leading care of seriously ill patients. This seemed possible since the nurses knew me as a critical care nurse and a teacher of critical-care nursing. Therefore, they may perceive me as a source of help, advice and expertise. I was also aware that nurses on this ward had called on colleagues in intensive care previously to help when they felt unable to cope with the acuity of illness and level of care needed. I anticipated that it might cause some conflict for me as a researcher and as a nurse. To stand back and refuse to intervene or share knowledge in a situation could be seen as a failure to act in the best interests of the patient and as a breach of my code of professional conduct. However, to intervene might have significantly affected the nurses' actions under observation. This would break from the idea of naturally occurring data sought by qualitative researchers, and I feared that the findings of my study might be affected by my intervention with patients.

No amount of clear communication of 'why you are there' can ever hope to prevent dilemmas of this nature. The responsibility one has to the patient and to fellow nurses with whom one interacts cannot be simply put to one side by stating 'today I am here only as a researcher'. This is because, when things go awry, you are *in* the situation as a participant observer. In my research, the whole focus of the study was about when things go awry.

My initial attempts at observation confirmed my fears: that being around when patients became seriously ill made it difficult not to participate in a way which significantly directed the actions of the nurses and the way the situation progressed. I was asked to help and for my opinion about patients.

As a result, my data-collection strategy was revised. Extensive participant observation was abandoned in favour of less extensive *ad hoc* observation of the ward followed by in-depth open-ended interviews with nurses.

A further issue relates to the challenge of observing nursing as a nurse in the role of 'etic' researcher, that is as the 'outsider'. On initial attempts at observation, it became apparent that I was not a total outsider. I had worked in acute care before, albeit a number of years earlier. Because of this, much of what might have needed explanation to some researchers I already understood to some degree. For example, the nurses used the phrase 'going off'. By this I knew that they meant deteriorating severely. This made me question whether I was to some extent an insider looking at situations from an 'emic' perspective.

During the study, I repeatedly returned to the texts I had read about ethnography and in particular the concepts of 'etic' and 'emic'. At the outset, it was my idealistic belief that it was possible for me to fully understand the approach I was adopting and to employ it in quite a rule-governed way. Experience of attempting this type of study is an invaluable way of learning about the research approach. With experience, I concluded that a research approach is more like a set of ideas and principles that need adaptation, refinement and an open-minded stance by the researcher in order that they can be applied in a range of situations.

Undertaking research is about learning. Not just learning about your subject but also about the approach you are employing and, most challengingly, learning about yourself. My reflection, experience and further reading helped me to understand and apply more usefully the notions of emic and etic in my study. This was achieved by refining my view of these perspectives and why they are important for the researcher to adopt. The whole point of adopting an outsider's perspective is to observe what people actually do. This can then be compared with what people say that they do. Thus, even if I am a nurse studying nursing, by observing what people do rather than relying completely on what they say I can still bring an etic perspective to the study. This is not to say that people attempt to intentionally deceive researchers in their descriptions of what they do. However, the way they describe what they do, the meaning they derive from it and the emphasis they place on some occurrences may lead the researcher to have a different understanding from that which one can arrive at through a blend of observation and participants' accounts. The right balance of observation and interview will probably be different in each study.

However, in finding the right balance, the aim is to explore both emic and etic perspectives and in doing so compare each with the other in order that any complexities, contradictions and paradoxes are exposed and made more understandable.

A final challenge was managing the study within the time constraints. In the fieldwork period of three months, I managed to perform seven interviews. If I had gone along with my original strategy of observation followed by interviews of those observed, I would not have managed anywhere near as many. This would have severely limited the data collected and the perspective gained. Savage (1995), who performed a larger-scale ethnographic study of acute-care wards, used participant observation but also experienced only limited success. Again, the constraint was time. He writes: 'I was unable to undertake the kind of prolonged fieldwork that characterises orthodox anthropology.'

This also limited the scope of data collection and perspectives gained. The main fieldwork was in the form of in-depth open-ended interviews, which are the ethnographer's most important data-gathering technique.

## How I chose the study sample

Because the study was part of a master's degree dissertation, resources, researcher experience and time were more limited than they might have been in larger-scale funded research. These impositions were key factors in the decision to undertake a study of one ward as a case study rather than several wards as a more wide-scale ethnography.

Initially, I had a naive belief that an ideal ward for study should be identified. The attributes of the ideal ward included such characteristics as being relatively stable. By this I mean not in the midst of some structural, managerial or staffing upheaval. A further criterion was that the ward regularly had patients who were critically ill, either pre-transfer to intensive care, post-transfer from intensive care or who were critically ill and being nursed on the ward on an ongoing basis.

I approached the senior nurse of a local intensive care unit (selected for convenience) and asked for data on the ward that received most patients from and referred most patients to the intensive care unit. I then approached the director of nursing services and the nurse manager for the surgical unit where this ward was situated in order to gain permission for the study and to discuss the suitability of the ward for study. While Ethical Committee approval was not sought, written permission from the director of nursing for the hospital was given.

Perhaps because of my etic perspective and naivety about the state of acute-ward services, I was unaware that my initial criterion of stability was rather idealistic and that the ward caring for the most critically ill patients was also the ward with the least stability in many ways. This was the beginning of my reflexivity in realizing my assumptions as an outsider.

Because of my intent to study the case in a naturalistic environment rather than an outsider's ideal environment, I decided to study the busy surgical ward that I initially thought was in a state of upheaval. Further details about the nature of the ward are given later in the chapter. For the purposes of the study, the pseudonym of 'Davy Ward' was used.

As is customary in ethnography, I did not have a preset idea of the sample to interview, which eventually totalled seven qualified nurses from Davy Ward. As is also typical, I began selecting participants to interview using a fairly informal and pragmatic strategy. As I introduced myself to the ward staff (many of whom already knew me to some extent), I explained my study and gave written information and asked about the willingness of staff to be interviewed and the practical possibilities of interviewing staff on days that I had set aside for fieldwork.

Decisions regarding whom to interview were made using a *judgemental sampling* technique, as well as simply who was willing and available for interview on the allocated fieldwork days. Fetterman (1998) describes judgemental sampling as ethnographers relying on their judgement about the most appropriate members of the culture based on the research question. An attempt was made to gain a range of perspectives from staff of different clinical grades, educational levels, levels of experience and from day and night duty in the hope that this would give a richer and more holistic view. Many details were recorded about each nurse participating – for example, age, clinical grade, years of experience, education level and years working on Davy Ward. However, it was not an aim of the study to compare and contrast the information given by the different nurses or to draw conclusions based on assumptions about their grade, age or any other factor. The details were merely used to inform future judgements about sampling in order to avoid a predominantly junior or senior perspective, for example.

The seven interviews were performed over a three-month period, and even this small number proved difficult because of the staffing levels and workload. It was often unsafe to take staff away from the ward on busy shifts, of which there were very many. Thus, to impose a rigid list of who to interview would not have allowed the flexibility in interview scheduling that took place. As it was, many of the interviews were not performed on allocated fieldwork days but on my days off, *ad hoc* annual leave days and in the middle of the night prior to a full working day.

# How I analysed the data

The interviews generated 101 A4 pages of typed, single-spaced transcript. I undertook the majority of the transcribing, with transcription of excerpts from each interview also being undertaken by a colleague in an attempt to ensure accurate representations of the spoken word in the text of the transcript.

The reason I undertook the majority of the transcribing was that I experienced great difficulty in finding someone willing to transcribe for what I considered a reasonable fee. One distinct disadvantage of performing the transcribing was that it was very time-consuming. Each interview, which averaged an hour, took around eight to ten hours to transcribe. However, in doing the transcribing myself, the only limitation was my own time, and the project was not held up through waiting for others. If I had undertaken the whole process myself, I could have made erroneous assumptions about what was meant in the spoken word and misrepresented this in the transcript. However, I asked a colleague to listen to what I considered to be the more ambiguous or difficult-to-hear aspects of the tapes and give an opinion of what the nurses were trying to communicate. A further method employed to facilitate accurate representation was to give copies of the transcripts back to the originating nurses and ask whether it was a true representation of what they had said. The most positive outcome of performing the transcribing myself was that during the process I began to be immersed in the data, as part of the analysis process.

Moore (2000) outlines some general principles for analysing qualitative textual data. These include the principle that analysis should be systematic but not rigid. The literature on such strategies and methods is vast and, as suggested by Moore, the importance of a system is paramount.

> You should adopt an organised approach, pursuing lines of enquiry and documenting your work as you go on (Moore 2000).

The systematic approach adopted in this study was an eclectic approach adapted from several published guides on the topic (Moore 2000, Benner et al. 1996, Burnard 1991). After much reading and reflection, I developed this eclectic approach out of pragmatic necessity. As one relatively inexperienced at analysing data of this type I needed an approach that was straightforward and simple to execute but that allowed for an exploration of ideas as well as an ability to retrace my steps in the process.

The stages in the data analysis process are as follows:

## Stage 1
Notes were made throughout the process of performing sequential interviews. Thus thoughts about the data were cultivated from the outset of

fieldwork (Moore 2000). These served as a way of noting impressions of the interview and ideas and theories to be explored in more depth later in the process.

## Stage 2
Transcripts of the interviews were made using a word-processor package (Microsoft Word for Windows 2000), and a general feel for the data was gained. Again, notes were made regarding salient themes or ideas and the process of becoming immersed in the data began (Moore 2000). The transcripts were aligned serially in a single document file and the pages numbered. Copies of individual interview transcripts were sent to each individual nurse interviewed. This was done in order that they could validate that what they had said or meant by their comments had been maintained during the transcription process.

## Stage 3
The text was read through and notes were made in the margins of the text. Rather than coding the text (Burnard 1991), it was named. Descriptive names were developed and broadly defined for aspects of the text seen as salient to the study focus (Benner et al. 1996). The process of naming and the changing of names was undertaken in order to get closer to the meaning in the text rather than focusing on marking the text using codes in a more distant way (Benner et al. 1996).

## Stage 4
A list of names was made, and the text was read again and again with the location of the named text being entered in brackets next to corresponding names. Thus, each name and brief description had bracketed locations of all the text given that specific name. As the names were given, broad headings were developed under which seemingly related portions of text were grouped together. At this stage, these were tentative groupings.

## Stage 5
When all text had been named, the names were worked through and repetitious or similar names were collapsed in order to reduce the number of descriptive names.

## Stage 6
Using the word-processor package, all the text was cut and pasted into categories according to its name. The page number from where it was cut was entered in brackets next to the text in order that its original source was identifiable. This was done so that if further exploration or clarification of

the portion of text were needed its original context and the nurse who said this could be referred to (Burnard 1991, Benner et al. 1996). This was possible because during Stage 1 all the interviews had been typed together in a single document. Thus pages 1 to 12 were from interview one, pages 13 to 24 were from interview two, and so on.

Stage 7
Selected respondents were asked to check the appropriateness of the naming system. They were asked whether comments they made during their interview had been appropriately named. This allowed for a validity check (Burnard 1991) to ensure that the meaning of their comments had been maintained and represented.

Stage 8
The writing-up process began, and the results of the analysis were related to and compared with the literature in order to further validate, challenge and compare the findings with the existing body of knowledge (Burnard 1991).

The data-analysis process initially resulted in five categories with various related themes arranged under each category. These were reworked and reflected upon and, although the five initial categories were retained, their names were changed as their content was analysed in relation to the conceptual framework (Figure 6.1). The findings are presented below.

# What were my findings?

The three central concepts of 'compatibility', 'relative advantage' and 'practical applicability' from the literature were evident in the interview data. Although these concepts were chosen as category headings, it was often impossible to separate the three concepts within these categories. Data from the interview transcripts are presented throughout the chapter, in the form of verbatim quotes, to substantiate each category. The implication of the findings is discussed within each of the sections below.

## Context

Conversations with the surgical manager and ward staff and attempts at participant observation early in the study revealed background information about the ward and the context of nursing. Some salient details are reported here.

The ward was a 34-bed acute surgical ward. It is given the pseudonym here of Davy Ward. Eight consultants had beds on Davy Ward performing a range of specialist surgery. For numerous reasons, patients on Davy Ward were generally having increasingly complex and extensive surgery increasing their dependency and morbidity and giving the ward a reputation for being one of the busiest wards in the hospital.

At the time of the study (October to December 2000), the G grade sister was on long-term sick leave and the F grade sister had recently left. A G grade sister from an adjacent ward was overseeing the ward but was soon to retire. One of the E grade nurses was appointed as an F grade towards the end of the study.

All the nurses interviewed expressed perceptions that many patients were 'highly dependent' and 'seriously ill'. The nurses' experiences of caring for these patients was the focus of the interviews.

> **Nurse 5**: We seem to always have had, since the summer, two bays full who are what I would say are medium dependency or high dependency patients.

The dependency of the patients seemed to be related to their care needs and the severity of their illness.

> **Nurse 5**: Recently, a gentleman was on the ward and he was very ill ... He was overloaded, with fluid, grossly overloaded – about ten litres or more positive balance; he'd got a low albumin. He was breathless. He was shutdown.

Many patients were undeniably very ill, and without a high dependency unit within the hospital these patients had to be cared for in either the ICU or the ward. It has been recommended that patients should be classified according to the severity of their illness and need for support rather than by location (DoH 2000). However, staffing to support this dependency was inadequate.

> **Nurse 2**: I can't have one nurse looking after 12 patients when they are that ill.

This has not been ignored in the reviews of critical care. However, the issue of understaffing seems to have been eclipsed in many instances by a focus on the need for education and training.

> Ward staff cannot take on higher-dependency patients unless they are trained and supported (Audit Commission 1999).

However, it is important to look beyond calls for training and examine the context in which these nurses will attempt to learn and apply this in practice. The high workload and lack of staff to undertake this work was evident throughout the interviews. The result of this seems to be two-fold. First of all, there was a lack of time to care adequately for the patients – not just those who are critically ill but also the rest of the patients on the ward.

> **Nurse 4**: It was just the time element; having the time to give the care she needed without compromising anyone else.

Secondly, there is the issue that even those who might have the right knowledge and skills to care for the critically ill do not have time to use them so they have limited 'practical applicability'.

> **Nurse 5**: What's worrying is not having the time to use the knowledge and skills. But I mean we do do it and I'm not saying that we are always in that sort of state. But that is what it is often like on here. Bay 1 and 2 are sometimes just beyond what we can cope with.

The application of theory to practice is seen as the acid test of the success of education (Jordan 2000). The notion of 'practical applicability' refers to the extent to which learning outcomes can be implemented. However, to consider this concept as a measure of successful education or even to judge the quality or appropriateness of the education in relation to its impact in practice is simplistic. This is because it would appear that there is inadequate time to apply critical-care knowledge and skills to the situation and decide on an appropriate course of action.

The NHS Plan (DoH 2001) promises 'more staff' and 'more time'. However, meanwhile perhaps the 'sub-optimal care' described by McQuillan et al. (1998) is related to the lack of time and staff on acute wards. Nurses described letting patients down.

> **Nurse 5**: That is what really worries me – that somebody who's just had routine surgery will just be completely neglected because you are dealing with high-dependency patients.

There seems little recognition in the literature of the nursing impact on seriously ill patients, with McQuillan et al. (1998) and NCEPOD (1999) focusing on medical practice. The nurses on Davy Ward, however, seemed acutely aware of their contribution, potential contribution and often, because of staffing, inability to make contributions.

> Once we acknowledge the pervasive informal nursing role of frontline quality monitoring, managing breakdown, system repair and team building, we can build in supports and sanctions for nursing performance of this role (Benner et al. 1999).

This role seems underplayed in the larger scheme of modernizing critical care. One of very few comments regarding this in the literature was made by Youngs (1998) in a letter to the editor of the *British Medical Journal*:

> We now seem to rely on the ward nurses to call the 'physiology police' but with more than eight patients per trained nurse on the medical and surgical wards, detection of something physiologically abnormal is not reliable. I am sure this hospital is not unique in this situation. To have any chance of improving the quality of acute medical care on general wards there must be either fewer patients or more medical and nursing staff.

The inadequate staffing levels did not only seem to affect the patients but also the carers. Working on the ward was seen as stressful, even frightening.

> **Nurse 5**: I mean really we should have [more staff] we are not just here to run around. It really worries me sometimes, I mean we've got to live with that [failures in care] then haven't we?

The emphasis placed on recruitment and retention in critical care documents (DoH 2000, Audit Commission 1999) and the proposed link between burnout and nurse attrition (Nolan et al. 1998, Williams et al. 1998, Price Waterhouse 1988) mean that the stress of nursing on wards seems a very important issue for managers, educators and policy makers to consider.

Being busy limits practical application of learning. However, one experienced nurse gave an interesting perspective on this issue. Her comments support the value of educating staff who are 'very busy' and highlight the way in which there *can* be 'relative advantage'.

> **Nurse 2**: I would say it's being busy and having to cut corners that sometimes makes using such knowledge advantageous. If you're cutting corners, you need to know which ones you can cut safely.

It seems that there is a paradox here. The nurses claim that there is no time to apply knowledge and skills, yet this nurse claims that, if applied, they might buy time for the nurse not least because of preventing patient deterioration.

## Compatibility

'Compatibility' has been defined as the degree to which learning is compatible with the needs of the nurse and the organization. 'Needs' might be seen to exist because there is a lack of knowledge and skill in an aspect of practice that offers 'relative advantage'. However, for such aspects of practice to be 'compatible' they have to be congruent with the way nurses perceive their role. Within this category illumination of compatible education was achieved. However, the complexities of compatibility as a concept in clinical practice were also highlighted.

Patient assessment and monitoring were prevalent themes. It emerged from descriptions of experiences. Thus, knowledge and skills of assessment were seen to offer 'relative advantage' and 'practical applicability' as well as being 'compatible'. In some instances, the nurses described noticing salient abnormalities:

> **Nurse 2**: I came on the late shift to find him semi-comatose. His respirations were about ten and his oxygen saturations were 78%. His chest was dreadful with fluid you could hear [without a stethoscope] ... and the drain was full of air so he had obviously perforated [his bowel].

On other occasions assessment did not include findings the nurses 'came across'. Rather, the assessment and monitoring were more deliberate and routine.

> **Nurse 4**: We had to do regular observations on her and especially saturations because they kept dropping.

Assessment was a prerequisite for action. The action may have been intervening autonomously or calling for help or review by another health professional.

> **Nurse 5**: I alerted the doctors to his predicament in the first place. I mean, we were monitoring him and they wouldn't have known anything about it if we hadn't told them ... we were doing his urine output regularly and his blood pressure etc.

Potential 'relative advantage' was also evident where lack of assessment led to deterioration.

> **Nurse 7**: Well, he'd got a central line in. He'd got an infection from it – no observations done, no temperature done, so we'd not picked up on it.

A range of published literature reports on the 'relative advantage' of nursing assessment and identification of significant abnormal physiology in ward patients. This supports the 'compatibility' of assessment with nursing (Cioffi 2000, Russell 2000, Benner et al. 1999, Gibson 1997, Daffurn et al. 1994, Franklin and Mathew 1994, Benner 1984).

Assessment was one example from a range of aspects of practice, the full listing of which is beyond the scope of this chapter. However, a number of other aspects of practice were less clear-cut. The perspective gained from the study highlighted the complexities that might be experienced in attempting to encapsulate compatible skills and knowledge in educational interventions, as well as the conflict that nurses face in daily practice.

The complexities of including compatible educational programme content were made real when it seemed that the nurses experienced internal conflict over what was and what was not their role. It seemed that some of the nurses exhibited an ideal and a contradictory real view of what caring for the critically ill necessitated in terms of their role. Nurses described thinking that in an ideal world they should not have to advise junior doctors about what to prescribe but the reality was they had to, and this caused internal conflict.

There was also conflict between nurses and other staff about their role. An example of this was where pharmacists gave nurses the explicit message that nurses should be checking doctors' prescriptions. This was not limited to pharmacists; medical staff also gave out similar messages; however, some medical staff also told the nurses 'that is my job, not yours'.

Other examples were discussed during the interviews and offer an interesting perspective on the notion of compatibility and role perception. If nurses are to be prepared for critical care, their role and scope of practice needs to be represented in the educational content. That is, education needs to be compatible. However, with conflicting messages over what nurses should and should not contribute to care, the issue of compatibility seems complex and contradictory.

Benner (1984) discusses nurses believing that drug-prescribing errors should not happen. They were seen as system failures. They were the ones who often noticed such errors and advised the physicians on corrections. But they did not talk with pride about this aspect of their role. This is perhaps the paradox of making a difference but feeling ashamed about it, or denying its legitimacy as part of nursing.

> For the sake of economy, we need to avoid documenting the obvious and agreed-upon issues and focus our search on the confusing and conflicting ones (Benner 1984).

The Department of Health has related the importance of competencies over professional boundaries in the delivery of safe, efficient and effective critical-care services (DoH 2000). Earlier, in *Clinical Governance* (DoH 1999), they also argued that organizations in which quality is likely to thrive are characterized by a determination to break down barriers between professional groups. This is no easy task when beliefs about what nurses should and should not do are so contradictory and so deeply entrenched (Cutler 2000a, 2000b).

## Collaboration

The essence of this category is about the nature of collaboration in the process of caring for the critically ill. A large part of nursing the critically ill on Davy Ward seemed to involve working with medical staff. However, features of this resonate with those from the last category with nurses discussing the way reality did not fit with their ideology that 'doctors should know' and that nurses should not have to advise them.

Nurses talked frequently about the lack of knowledge and skill of Pre-registration House Officers (PRHOs) and Senior House Officers (SHOs). This was significant for them because these were often their first, or only, line of medical support when a patient became seriously ill.

> **Nurse 3**: So when you tell a doctor that the reading [central venous pressure] has changed, they say 'Oh right – what should it be?' They don't even know.

There was an evident perception of relative advantage here. The advantage being that, even if a doctor does not, the nurses may know and the sharing of knowledge under such circumstances may benefit the patient.

Benner et al.'s (1996) chapter discussing the nurse-physician relationship, and earlier work (Benner 1984, Stein 1967) acknowledges how the nurse provides a back-up system for deficits in medical knowledge and practice. Despite an ideology that 'doctors should know', they too begin as novices, and they can learn a great deal from experienced nurses, but only if they collaborate (Cutler 2000b).

It was apparent on Davy Ward that nurses often made a difference in the care of the critically ill by advising and teaching PRHOs. However, there is an interesting paradox here. It seems that nurses on Davy Ward were aware of the lack of knowledge amongst PRHOs. They were also aware that in sharing their knowledge and experience with the PRHOs both the doctors and the patients benefited. However, this was strongly at odds with their belief that 'doctors should know'.

It is also worth noting that the advising and teaching of PRHOs by nurses was part of normal practice for more senior or experienced nurses, not novices. In the process of the study, it became apparent that the things that made a real difference ('relative advantage') were evident in more experienced nurses. Preparing nurses for practice, one could argue, is not just about teaching aspects of practice. It is also about the awareness of the paradoxes of reality and may involve challenging ideologies, being mindful of experience and how role perception and the wisdom of nurses changes with experience.

Looking at this issue from a different perspective, one could argue that nurses should not have to teach doctors, and that from the first category

('Context') it was apparent that they had too much to do already. Another answer might be having more senior doctors on hand to help educate the PRHOs and review the more seriously ill patients. However, in the case of the staff on Davy Ward, getting *any* doctors to perform timely reviews of patients was often difficult. This was another feature of the collaboration, and lack of collaboration, that took place. The doctors often failed to review patients that the nurses thought were deteriorating.

> **Nurse 2** : The drain was full of air so he had obviously perforated [his bowel]. It had been relayed to the doctors in the morning about ten o'clock that he wasn't well, and at four o'clock we finally got him reviewed by a senior registrar who then called in the relatives and said that he wasn't for resuscitation.

The publication of McQuillan et al.'s (1998) study on sub-optimal ward care was followed by letters to the *British Medical Journal*'s editor; one noted:

> nursing staff on general medical and surgical wards identify a significant number of patients whom they feel warrant admission to a high dependency or intensive care unit. Worryingly, most of such patients identified during this audit were not reviewed regularly by experienced medical staff (Ringrose and Garrard 1998).

Benner et al. (1996) identify abilities of nurses that tended to facilitate physician review. The abilities include having a strong clinical grasp and judgement of the situation, knowing the doctors and having developed relationships with them and being skilled in making a case that the patient needs review. Such abilities should perhaps be a standard part of criticalcare nurse education.

In the light of difficulties in summoning doctors to review critically ill patients, the nurses on Davy Ward described how they often stepped outside the medical prescription or acted first and told the doctor later.

> **Nurse 1**: Well, say, for example, a patient comes back from theatre and they are hypotensive and their oxygen saturations have dropped, and we would put some oxygen on and speed their drip up and then we get in touch with a doctor.

The nurses described the relative advantage this brought to care and the need to know when to step outside the medical prescription. Clauses in the Code of Professional Conduct (UKCC 1992) centre on ensuring no harm comes to the patient via action or omission. In the complexity of real life on busy hospital wards this double-edged sword put the nurse in a very difficult position. Acting outside the medical prescription and making a positive difference in doing so is not a skill that one might expect from a novice nurse. This again seems to support the notion that teaching this ability is extremely difficult (Benner et al. 1999) not least because it may well have low compatibility with the role perception of novice nurses.

Educational preparation for these abilities requires the educator to take account of the complexities of practice and the trajectory of learning and experience that nurses might travel. Much of the relative advantage discussed in this category challenges the ideology that 'doctors should know' and highlights the subtle but important nuances of clinical nursing that lie outside what might be thought of as the traditional and legitimate role of the nurse (Cutler 2000b).

### Relative advantage

'Relative advantage' has been defined as the degree to which the learned material is perceived as better than that which it supersedes. This category focuses on perspectives on how and why knowledge is empowering in practice and, in contrast, how lack of it was perceived as disempowering for the nurses. This category also focuses on nurses' awareness of a lack of knowledge and skill, as well as a lack of awareness since these gave an additional perspective on relative advantage.

One nurse demonstrated how her knowledge of falling oxygen saturations helped inform her clinical judgement about a seriously ill patient.

> **Nurse 4:** We had to do regular observations on her and especially saturations because they kept dropping, and obviously if they drop – why are they dropping? Did she need suction? Has she got her humidified oxygen on properly? If a junior nurse was there and the sats dropped, they would probably think 'her sats have dropped – let's get a doctor' and, through no fault of their own – because I've been there – they don't think about what could be wrong.

To call a doctor in the case of falling oxygen saturations might seem appropriate action. However, in the context of Davy Ward, because of the difficulties of getting timely responses from doctors, to act first and tell the doctor later might be more appropriate. It was also argued by the nurses that autonomous actions by them, for example performing endobronchial suction, might preclude the need to have a doctor attend at all. The relative advantage of clinical judgement is obviously in deciding what the problem is and deciding on an appropriate course of action.

Clinical judgement is not just about knowing the facts of oxygen saturation, what is normal for example; it is much more than that (Schon 1987). It requires reasoning about open-ended clinical situations that might present as unique cases (Benner et al. 1999). The literature on clinical judgement portrays a picture of a complex interplay of cognitive processes with the 'messyness' of reality (Schon 1987). It could be argued that such abilities are very different to the behavioural competencies some might assume are the goal of the mandates outlined in the *Comprehensive Critical Care* document (DoH 2000).

In this sense, relative advantage, through clinical judgement, offers a different perspective on practical applicability. It might be seen not just as a characteristic of the taught/learned material but also as a concept that is related to the *way* in which the material is taught and learned. Without the opportunity and support to utilize learned material in practice, it may have no practical applicability. It may remain an abstract cognitive item, for example – 'normal oxygen saturations are above 95%'. Benner et al. (1999) note that much of clinical learning about complex clinical situations is acquired 'on the job' and is taught informally by preceptors. The challenge in education is to bring this marginalized learning into planned educational programmes (Benner et al. 1999, Schon 1987).

The nurses discussed knowledge around a range of subjects that they perceived offered relative advantage as well as compatibility and practical applicability.

> **Nurse 2**: Knowledge about fluid overload and fluid challenges. I think fluid challenges are important to know about because there is a fine line between a fluid challenge being beneficial and the patient becoming overloaded and needing Frusemide, and that happens a lot on our ward.

All the nurses discussed fluid management. This has been acknowledged as a serous issue in the care of seriously ill ward patients, not least because it has been shown to cause preventable morbidity and mortality (NCEPOD 1999). Hence, there is an obvious relative advantage. Other areas included physiology, disease, pharmacology, family care and more technical aspects, such as care of central venous lines.

In some cases, nurses were aware that they had a skill or knowledge deficit:

> **Nurse 2**: We do have patients on here that are really ill at times, and it goes beyond our knowledge and for somebody to come along and say 'you need to be doing this' or 'watch for this' or 'have you checked so and so?'. That would be lovely.

A notion underpinning the research approach as an outsider was that to make assumptions about what nurses needed to know or be able to do might potentially lead to a misinformed curriculum. However, to ask, and simply rely on, the nurses' perceived needs might overlook skills or knowledge that they were not aware of. This phenomenon has been referred to as 'secondary ignorance', that is 'They do not know what they do not know' (Benner et al. 1996). This was evident when one nurse was discussing central venous lines:

> **Nurse 3**: Well, there is only the sister who flushes them [central lines] because she's been on the course ... I don't know really – I'll probably learn it on this study day. At the minute, we just hope it is all right and just leave it alone.

This 'hope it is all right' approach is an indication of secondary ignorance.

In the paradox of not knowing about one's limitations, an outsider is perhaps required to give additional insight. However, if all curriculum content was decided by an outsider, one might not take account of the context in which learning has to be implemented. Or indeed acknowledge the impediments to clinical application. Outsiders also suffer ignorance in that they do not know about the context of insiders' practice.

In defence of ethnography, Boyle (1994) argues that the combination of emic and etic views side by side produce a 'third dimension' rounding out the ethnographic picture. It seems that the same could be said of the combination of insiders' and outsiders' perspectives on educational programme content, that they produce something more rounded and holistic than if either had chiefly informed the curriculum alone.

### An ideology of learning

This category focuses on evident ideologies about learning discussed by the nurses. Ideology here refers to ideal and abstract views (SOED 1973). It could be argued that these ideal and abstract views are important for educators to consider, since they allow some understanding of the perspective nurses may bring to teaching/learning interactions.

Very salient were the nurses' negative views of some formal education programmes they had undertaken. While commenting on a degree-level surgical-nursing course, one nurse related:

> **Nurse 1**: I didn't get out of it [the course] what I thought I'd get out of it. I expected too much of it I think ... I think it should focus more on physiological problems and the things we see on the ward, the things that happen with our patients. I think we should look at situations that arise, but we didn't.

Not all views expressed about formal education programmes were negative. However, many views indicated that the courses were not seen to lead to learning that offered practical applicability, compatibility and relative advantage. One nurse succinctly related this:

> **Nurse 7**: I come out and think, 'I have not learned anything from that'. You have got to be able to bring it back and apply it to what you are doing.

Such views are supported in the broader literature. *Integrating Theory and Practice in Nursing* (NHSE 1998) sought the views of all stakeholders in education and identified some key issues that require consideration in future educational planning. These included what was described as 'upward academic drift', which was similar to the perception of universities not being practice-orientated. The ability to provide educational support for learning in practice, the skills or practice component of education programmes diminishing and the question of whether nurse teachers should still practise clinical nursing were also thought to be key.

Some of these themes were echoed in the transcripts, for example the nurses expressed a belief in the value of clinical experience in learning. Nurses were asked how they had learned to care for critically ill patients.

> **Nurse 4**: I wouldn't really say I got anything from my nurse training. I know that sounds shocking coming out with that but ... I think mostly from just being on here.

Experience was valued by nurses, and lack of experience was seen to be a major factor related to a lack of clinical knowledge and abilities. However, the nurses did not reject teachers but rather expressed the view that they could be of great value in facilitating learning from practice in the clinical area. They also complained that this was not formally supported and that preceptorship was poor on Davy Ward. An experienced nurse said:

> **Nurse 1**: When nurses are newly qualified, I don't think they are well preceptored. I think they get thrown in.

It seems that there is a great potential to learn from the experience of caring for the critically ill (Benner et al. 1999), especially if this experience is augmented by sharing and analysing experiences with other nurses and educators. However, the relevant educators were mainly engaged in classroom-based teaching activities. The novices, who required most support and had most to learn with regard to critical care on the ward, were left to experience without adequate support.

The benefits of teachers returning to practice and supporting clinical learning have been outlined elsewhere (NHSE 1998, Glossop et al. 1999). However, at present there is little formal support for such endeavours. The paradox here, it could be argued, is that until those responsible for formulating and delivering nurse-education programmes are closer to practice, both geographically and ideologically, their approach may be at odds with those whom they wish to educate. In their over-reliance on classroom teaching, they may fail to deliver education that is informed by the clinical practice from which they are so far removed. The risk is that practical applicability, compatibility and relative advantage fail to feature highly enough in the formulation of course content and the orientation of formal learning experiences. Edmond suggests a growing realization of these issues: .

> Education for all practice disciplines is about to undergo a paradigm shift whereby the value of practical education and experience will be better understood, more rigorously analysed and integrated with professional knowledge in the constructions of personal professional knowledge and identity (Edmond 2001).

The future will enable valid judgements about this prophetic assertion.

## Conclusions

This study did not set out to confirm that the nurses on the ward would like to know, for example, how to safely care for central venous catheters. It was taken for granted that such elements of knowledge would be useful, yet it was assumed that there is much more to know about the everyday reality of nursing the critically ill. The aims of this study were to develop a deeper understanding of the clinical context of learners' practice, because of a belief that it would enable the development of more congruent, relevant and applicable educational content.

Despite espousing the idea that ward-based critical-care nursing is complex, it is now acknowledged that some rather simplistic assumptions informed the researcher's previous perspective. Amongst them was the idea that 'practical applicability', 'compatibility' and 'relative advantage' (Rogers and Shoemaker 1971) were simple concepts that would emerge from the data as monoliths informing future educational practice and the content of educational programmes. What was discovered instead was a range of very complex issues, such as discussed above, as well as some interesting paradoxes.

The paradox of 'practical applicability' related to an evident perception that there was inadequate time to apply learning in practice. However, applying learning in practice, in relation to the critically ill, might actually buy some time through prevention of deterioration and knowing what could safely be omitted from care at very busy times, for example.

The paradox in relation to 'compatibility' centred on the contradictory messages that came from nurses, as well as other members of the multidisciplinary team, about their perceived roles and responsibilities with the critically ill. Nurses even contradicted themselves about what they believed and understood their role to be. As a result, this made the issue of what they needed to know and apply in practice quite complex.

A paradox in relation to 'collaboration' was that nurses expressed the opinion that they should not have to advise and guide junior doctors – 'they should know'. But at the same time they acknowledged that in reality they often *had* to advise and that developing certain types of knowledge would put them in a better position to do this. This was a paradox of the ideal scenario versus what the real world demanded of them in order to keep patients safe.

The paradox in relation to 'relative advantage' was focused on the difficulty of discovering what knowledge and judgements would offer relative advantage to the practitioners. Insiders may suffer from what has been called 'secondary ignorance' (Benner et al. 1996). That is, 'They do not know what they do not know.' Conversely, outsiders may not understand the complexity and paradoxes within the local setting and may make assumptions about what can be transferred from the ICU or high-dependency unit (HDU) setting, for example. This highlights the lack of depth and maturity that ward-based critical care faces. Greater study, curriculum development and evaluation are required before such assumptions and ignorance can be overcome. However, this may be made all the more difficult because of the final paradox.

The paradox in relation to 'an ideology of learning' is about the different values and beliefs that practitioners and educators, outside the hospital culture, seem to espouse in their attempts to improve the situation. Clearly, each may fail to see the validity of the other's perspective, and the situation may see little rapid improvement. This is particularly the case when clinicians put little faith in university-based education, accusing university teachers of 'upward academic drift' and when university teachers perceive that a lack of an application of learning is the fault of the learners (NHSE 1998). Such complexities and paradoxes present major challenges.

> The world is so awash in paradox and contradiction that each of us is forced to choose on a daily basis whether we are going to deal with the simultaneous validity of both sides of the same continuum or whether we are going to deny one side or the other (Wacker and Taylor 2000).

I would argue that the first step in dealing with these paradoxes and the issues they raise is acknowledging that the paradoxes exist. The presence of such paradoxes, however, cannot be assumed to exist in all staff and in all acute-ward areas. It is important that certain acknowledgements are made about the study findings here – primarily that this study was small scale and, in being a case study, was a study of the singular (Bassey 1999). One may be justified in arguing that because of this the findings cannot be generalized. However, Bassey (1999) writes of 'fuzzy generalisations' that he explains are statements with built-in uncertainty. This is not built in as an admission that the findings of case-study research are frail. Rather, it acknowledges that the complex realities of everyday interactions and complex social phenomena cannot always be manipulated and predicted. Understanding their complexity and contradictory nature is paramount.

Despite best efforts to describe the intricacies of the study, it is neither desirable nor possible, because of the nature of reality, to reproduce the study. Thus, a major limitation is that the study stands alone as a snap-shot of Davy Ward through the researcher's eyes and the words of the nurses at the time of the study. Since the study, two welcome changes have been seen: a critical-care outreach team has been established and plans for a high-dependency unit have been accepted.

# References

Audit Commission (1999) Critical to Success: the place of efficient and effective critical care services within the acute hospital. London: Audit Commission.

Bassey M (1999) Case Study Research in Educational Settings. Buckingham: Open University Press.

Benner P (1984) From Novice to Expert: excellence and power in clinical nursing practice. Menlo Park, Ca: Addison-Wesley.

Benner P, Tanner CA, Chelsa CA (1996) Expertise in Nursing Practice: caring, clinical judgement and ethics. New York: Springer Publishing Company.

Benner P, Hooper-Kyriakidis S, Stannard D (1999) Clinical Wisdom and Interventions in Critical Care: a thinking in action approach. Philadelphia, Pa: WB Saunders.

Boyle J (1994) Styles of ethnography. In Morse JM (ed.) Critical Issues in Qualitative Research Methods. Thousand Oaks, Ca: Sage.

Burnard P (1991) A method of analysing interview transcripts in qualitative research. Nurse Education Today 11(6): 461-466.

Burns N, Grove SK (1993) The Practice of Nursing Research: conduct critique and utilization (second edition). Philadelphia, Pa: WB Saunders.

Cioffi J (2000) Recognition of patients who require emergency assistance: a descriptive study. Heart and Lung 29(4): 262-268.

Cutler LR (2000a) Reflection on diagnosing as a nurse in ITU. Nursing in Critical Care 5(1): 22-28.

Cutler LR (2000b) The diagnostic domain of nursing. Nursing in Critical Care 5(2): 59-61.

Daffurn K, Lee A, Hillman K et al. (1994) Do nurses know when to summon emergency assistance? Intensive and Critical Care Nursing 10(2): 115-120.

Department of Health (DoH) (1999) Clinical Governance: quality in the new NHS. London: Department of Health.

Department of Health (DoH) (2000) Comprehensive Critical Care: a review of adult critical care services. London: Department of Health.

Department of Health (DoH) (2001) The NHS Plan: a plan for investment, a plan for reform. London: Department of Health.

Edmond CB (2001) A new paradigm for practice education. Nurse Education Today 21(4): 251-259.

Ellis L, Crookes P (1998) Philosophical and theoretical underpinnings of research. In Crookes PA, Davies S (eds.) Research into Practice. Edinburgh: Baillière Tindall.

Fetterman DM (1998) Ethnography: step by step (second edition). London: Sage.

Franklin C, Mathew J (1994) Developing strategies to prevent in-hospital cardiac arrest: analyzing responses of physicians and nurses in the hours before the event. Critical Care Medicine 22(2): 244-247.

Germain C (1979) The Cancer Unit: an ethnography. Wakefield, Ma: Nursing Resources.

Gibson JME (1997) Focus of nursing in critical and acute settings: prevention or cure? Intensive and Critical Care Nursing 13(3):163-166.

Glossop D, Hoyles A, Lees S et al. (2000) Benefits of nurse teachers returning to practice. British Journal of Nursing 8(6): 394-400.

Hargreaves DH (1996) Teaching as a research-based profession: possibilities and prospects. Teacher Training Agency Annual Lecture 1996. London: Teacher Training Agency.

Hunt M (1991) Qualitative research. In Cormack DFS (ed.) The Research Process in Nursing (second edition). London: Blackwell Scientific Publications.

Jordan S (2000) Educational input and patient outcomes: exploring the gap. Journal of Advanced Nursing 31(2): 461-471.

LeCompte MD, Schensul JJ (1999) Designing and Conducting Ethnographic Research. Walnut Creek, Ca: Altamira Press.

Leininger M (1985) Ethnography and ethnonursing: models and modes of qualitative data analysis. In Leininger M (ed.) Qualitative Research Methods in Nursing. New York: Grune & Stratton.

MacLeod Clark J, Hockey L (1989) Research for Nursing. Chichester: John Wiley and Sons.

Mathews L, Venables A (1998) Critiquing ethical issues in published research. In Crookes PA, Davies S (eds.) Research into Practice. Edinburgh: Baillière Tindall.

McQuillan P, Allan A, Taylor B et al. (1998) Confidential enquiry into quality of care before admission to intensive care. British Medical Journal 316(7148): 1853-1858.

Moore N (2000) How to do Research: the complete guide to designing and managing research projects (third edition). London: Library Association Publishing.

Morse JM (1991) Qualitative Health Research. London: Sage.

National Confidential Enquiry into Perioperative Deaths (NCEPOD) (1999) Extremes of Age: the 1999 report of the national confidential enquiry into perioperative deaths. London: NCEPOD.

National Health Service Executive (NHSE) (1998) Integrating Theory and Practice in Nursing: a report commissioned by the chief nursing officer/director of nursing. London: Department of Health.

Nolan M, Lundh U (1998) Ways of knowing in nursing and healthcare practice. In Crookes PA, Davies S (eds.) Research into Practice. Edinburgh: Baillière Tindall.

Nolan M, Broen J, Naughton M et al. (1998) Developing nursing's future role 2: nurses' job satisfaction and morale. British Journal of Nursing 7(17): 1044-1048.

Price Waterhouse (1988) Nurse Retention and Recruitment: a matter of priority. London: Price Waterhouse.

Ringrose T, Garrard C (1998) Doctors don't review patients that nurses identify as highly dependent. British Medical Journal 318(7175): 52.

Rogers EM, Shoemaker FF (1971) Communication of Innovations. New York: The Free Press.

Russell S (2000) Continuity of care after discharge from ICU. Intensive Care Nursing 15(8): 497-500.

Savage J (1995) Nursing Intimacy: an ethnographic approach to nurse-patient interaction. London: Scutari Press.

Schon DA (1987) Educating the Reflective Practitioner. San Francisco, Ca: Jossey-Bass.

Seymour JE (2001) Critical Moments: death and dying in intensive care. Buckingham: Open University Press.

Shorter Oxford English Dictionary (SOED) (1973) Volume I. Oxford: Clarendon Press.

Stein LI (1967) The doctor-nurse game. Archives of General Psychiatry 16(6): 699-703.

Stern PN (1994) Eroding grounded theory. In Morse JM (ed.) Critical Issues in Qualitative Research Methods. Thousand Oaks, Ca: Sage.

Streubert HJ (1995) Ethnographic research approach. In Streubert HJ, Carpenter R (eds.) Qualitative Research in Nursing: advancing the humanistic imperative. Philadelphia, Pa: Lippincott.

Thorne SE (1991) Methodological orthodoxy in qualitative nursing research: analysis of the issues. Qualitative Health Research 1(2): 178-199.

United Kingdom Central Council for Nursing, Midwifery and Health Visiting (UKCC) (1992) Code of Professional Conduct. London: UKCC.

Wacker W, Taylor J (2000) The Visionary's Handbook. Oxford: Capstone.

Williams S, Michie S, Pattari S (1998) Improving the NHS Workforce: report of the partnership on health of the NHS workforce. London: The Nuffield Trust.

Youngs PJ (1998) Inadequate staffing means problems are missed. British Medical Journal 318(7175): 52.

# CHAPTER SEVEN
# Phenomenology

CHRIS BASSETT

## Introduction

This chapter considers the use of phenomenology as a useful research method for understanding better some of the hidden and personal issues that may be present in the health care relationship. The author, who is a nurse lecturer, has an abiding interest in the use of qualitative research methodologies in health care. This chapter describes phenomenology as a research method and as a philosophy, and offers it as a way forward in measuring the possible effectiveness in the counselling relationship. It is divided into two distinct parts: first, a discourse on the elements of the research method and, secondly, a description of a research study carried out into the nature of the caring relationship between nurses and their patients.

## Phenomenology as a research method

This chapter describes a research method that may be of use to the heath researchers in helping better understand the issues surrounding their work and, indeed, the actual effectiveness of the care they give. The first part of this section explores the methodology and the philosophical paradigm underpinning it; the second part considers some studies that used phenomenology as their method of enquiry.

### Theoretical framework

As with any inquiry, it is the way exploration is undertaken that is the key to its success or otherwise (Field and Morse 1985, Cormack 1991, Stevens et al. 1993, Parahoo 1997). What of researching issues such as health care? If we take the view that caring is an individual subjective interaction between two persons, it may be that an understanding and measurement of that process, and any movement within that process, go beyond the limits of conventional or quantitative research methods. It is arguably impossible to use traditional quantitative research methods to understand the complexity of human nature. People cannot be reduced to simple numbers, as might be the aim of quantitative research methods; we need a research method that originates from a different and person-centred paradigm, and this paper offers phenomenology as one possible way forward. The writer has used this methodology to increase understanding in nursing care and believes that this methodology may help researchers to explore the attitudes, feelings and beliefs of the person undertaking the caring process.

## Phenomenology

Phenomenology uses the lived experience of the participants; in this case, the participants of the counselling relationship. As such, it explores the feeling and beliefs of individuals involved in that relationship. Heidegger, in Jensen (1993), believed that experiencing the world around us is the same as caring for it. He spoke of '*stimmung*' or attunement; this attunement when focused upon care states that care gives an existential quality which gives meaning and rhythm to all experience. In order to understand as fully as possible the ways that persons undertake counselling, it is important to explore the life worlds of those persons. Drew (1989) suggests the life world consists of the 'social, practical, experiential: a taken-for-granted dimension' that can be frequently overlooked by researchers, particularly those who come from a positivist, reductionist perspective.

In order to help understand the ways that people interpret their individual worlds, a qualitative approach that is inductive (theory generating) is described. This methodology uses a phenomenological approach, which attempts to understand the human life world as the individual experiences it (Omery 1983).

Phenomenology is both a philosophy and a research method (Ray 1994). Imanuel Kant first described it in 1764, in a scientific context, as the study of 'phenomena' and 'noumena' (Cohen 1987). This was then usefully summarized by Roche:

> We do not experience the external world purely, as it were. Our sensory experience of it is always and everywhere structured in terms of the categories of space and time, which are not, themselves, derived from experience. Categorical-sensory knowledge is thus limited and bounded; it is not capable of direct access to the external world as it is itself. Man only knows the appearances of things, never the things in themselves: that is to say, he can only ever know 'phenomena' and never 'noumena' (Roche 1973).

Phenomenology is therefore the study of phenomena or the appearance of things. This chapter will now briefly consider the emergence of the phenomenological movement. This, it is hoped, will help place the epistemology of this methodology in context and introduce some of the key issues in terms of validity and rigour, and help underpin its choice as a possible method for this type of human study. The term phenomenology was first used in 1764 relating to a variety of contexts from religion to philosophy. But it was Immanuel Kant's theory of phenomenology that truly started the phenomenological movement. The term 'movement' is an accurate one in that it has undergone change and development both in its understanding and indeed usage. It is very interesting to follow its development and to understand the influences that shaped its life. Spiegelberg (1960) divided the movement into three distinct parts that he called: the preparatory phase, the German phase and the French phase.

## The preparatory phase

The preparatory phase was driven by Franz Brentano (1838–1916) and by his first prominent student Carl Stumpf (1848–1936). Brentano wanted to answer questions using philosophy that, in his view, organized religion could no longer answer. He was also concerned with making psychology truly scientific. Two of Brentano's central tenets were particularly key to the later phenomenologists. These were the concepts of inner perception and its value. He was also the first to discuss the concept of intentionality. Intentionality is the notion that everything that we consider to be psychical refers to an object; for example we cannot hear without a sound or we cannot believe without believing in something.

## The German phase

Edmund Husserl (1859–1938) and latterly Martin Heidegger (1889–1976) directed the German phase. Husserl studied under and later worked with both Brentano and Stumpf. Husserl took his idea of phenomenology through several important stages of development. The first phase saw him explore equally the objective and subjective elements of experience. Later it was subjectivity that dominated his philosophy and was considered to be the source of all objectiveness. Husserl, like Stumpf earlier, became particularly concerned with rigour, this concern in direct opposition to the growing pre-war German hostility towards science.

Following the First World War, Husserl redirected his work. He wanted to create a philosophy that would restore contact with deeper human concerns. He then truly rejected the positivist paradigm. A central part of his new radicalism related to the important emergence of the concept and practice of phenomenological reductionism. Reductionism in this sense relates not to positivistic oversimplification but to the desire to obtain pure and clear phenomena that can be obtained by a naive attitude to the subject or thing.

The purpose of this reduction is to aid critical examination before our pre-existing belief and understanding enters in. Husserl used the Greek term *epokhē* (epoch) for this concept. Reduction involves two stages. The first, eidetic reduction is reduction from facts to general essences. Husserl used the mathematical metaphor of bracketing for this suspension of belief. The second stage, phenomenological reduction proper, frees phenomena from all trans-phenomenal elements. (The 'epoch' in modern research terms now refers to the bracketing out of internal prejudices, prejudgements etc.)

As Husserl's career moved towards its final stages, two further important concepts emerged. These were as a direct influence of the growing band of followers that were interested in phenomenology. The first was 'intersubjectivity'. This concept declares that a so-called plurality of subjectivities exist that makes up a community which shares a common world. The second concept is that of the 'life world'. This concept identifies that our everyday experience is not immediately accessible to us. We take so much for granted that we do not see what surrounds us (Omery 1983).

The Husserlian tradition is concerned with the nature of knowledge and asks the epistemological question of 'how we know'. It emphasizes a return to reflective intuition to describe and clarify experience as it is lived and constituted in the consciousness. Husserl believed that the personal, individual reality of the researcher could be put aside when analysing the data, by bracketing or holding it in suspension, thus making the research valid and true from the research subject's own personal viewpoint. Without bracketing, the data will be contaminated with the researcher's preconceptions. Martin Heidegger was another philosopher who is associated with the phenomenological movement. He came to Husserl first as student then as assistant. Heidegger saw phenomenology as a new means of finding solutions. Heidegger never considered phenomenology as truly integral to his philosophy, which was concerned mainly with 'being' and 'time'. Later, Heidegger became involved with the Nazi movement and essentially drifted, perhaps not surprisingly, away from Husserl, who was a Jew. Heidegger suggested that everyone is a self-interpreting being, therefore existing hermeneutically, finding significance and meaning in their everyday world (Ray 1994). Heidegger, and later Gadamer, moved the philosophical debate from epistemology to ontology, which asks, 'What is it to be?' Ontology is concerned with a way of 'being' in a socio-historical world where the fundamental dimensions of human consciousness are expressed through language (Ray 1994).

'Hermeneutics' means interpretation. Gadamer (1989) developed Heidegger's views and suggested that 'truth' is not objective knowledge as might be believed within the positivist tradition; instead, it encompasses the experience of being human. Subjective reality is, therefore, a legitimate way to inform the interpretation of the human phenomenon, that is things cannot be separated from the experience of them, and interpretation can only make explicit what is already understood.

The predominant feature of ontological hermeneutic philosophy is the 'hermeneutic circle'. The three basic tenets of the circle are:

- That we come into the world with a background, which is given to us by our culture from birth and presents a way of understanding what is real for a person.
- Pre-understanding is our structure of 'being in the world' and means that we come to a position with a history and a story, which cannot be bracketed or suspended. It is always with us in the world.
- Co-constitution means that we are constructed by the world in which we live, and at the same time construct the world from our experience and background.

Nothing can be encountered without reference to a person's background understanding, from which any interpretations are made. According to Heidegger, in Ray (1994), understanding is a way of *being*, not a way of *knowing*, and our capacity to understand is rooted in our own definitions of 'being in and of the world' or '*Dasein*' (being already in the world).

The hermeneutic circle is essentially that understanding is made from a given set of structures that cannot be eliminated but can only be corrected or modified. The hermeneutic approach therefore does not just acquire new knowledge, rather that which is already understood comes to be interpreted. The central and key distinction between Husserlian and Heideggerian approaches to researcher conduct and position is that, unlike Husserl, Heidegger believed that presuppositions are not to be eliminated or suspended. He believed that these helped interpretation of meaning within the phenomenon.

**The French phase**

Phenomenology shifted base during the early part of the Second World War to France and, following the war, phenomenology has become the dominant philosophy in France. It was Gabriel Marcel (1889–1973), Jean-Paul Sartre (1905–1980) and Maurice Merleau-Ponty (1907–1961) who became the most prominent figures at this time. These three philosophers developed the concept of phenomenology beyond that of previous thinkers. For instance, Sartre, who was a novelist and playwright prior to his work as a philosopher, used the term 'existentialist' in preference to 'phenomenologist'. He stressed individuals' responsibility for the creation of their own world. Sartre's goal was to use the ideals surrounding phenomenology to understand and was more concerned with practice than he was with theory. Merleau-Ponty was more concerned with the rigour and methodological issues than his friend Sartre.

The key issues remain today the same as they did for the founding fathers of phenomenology. It is the essential search for understanding the phenomenon that is important to the phenomenologist. Social scientists wishing to fully understand things and events have adopted and adapted phenomenology as a response to the realization that phenomena need to be studied in context rather than in isolation (Omery 1983); this is particularly true in the study of personal attitudes and beliefs. The value of phenomenology is that it is a method that aids the understanding of the human experience – not exploring reality itself but what reality is *perceived* to be (Moustakas 1994). Although there are many ways of transforming experience into knowledge or understanding (which is what this study aims to do), phenomenology is considered as being a particularly effective means of doing so (Reinharz 1983). It captures the experience in a specific context and attempts to make explicit what is implicit (Oiler 1982).

This philosophy often corresponds with the practitioner's personal philosophy and values. The notion of co-constitution is a predominant feature in the philosophy and can enable the research method to focus on how the individual in counselling may interpret their 'being' in the context of the counselling relationship.

### The philosophy as a research method

The aim of the method underpinned by this philosophy is to uncover hidden phenomena and meanings, by interpreting frequently taken-for-granted shared practices and common meanings, or what is not immediately manifest in our intuiting, analysing and describing (Omery 1983). The researcher develops a philosophical understanding, to see what is otherwise concealed. Understanding is not about correct procedure but is found in the hermeneutic circle. This means that the researcher brings personal pre-understanding to the text since this cannot be bracketed out (Ray 1994). The researcher therefore participates in the interpretation process and making the data. This approach, as Knaack (1984) notes, is in contrast to the scientific method, where the researcher passively receives knowledge and is unconnected (or as unconnected as possible) with the object.

In phenomenological study, an attempt is made to understand another person's subjective experiences and feelings by study of their field of expression. The field of expression is made up of speech, expression, gestures and intonations (Bassett 1994). The process of understanding occurs, according to Thibodeau (1993), when 'simultaneity' occurs, that is the sensation that the streams of consciousness of both the researcher and the researched flow along a temporarily parallel path. The 'stream of consciousness' described by the research subjects is unique to them. Schutz (1967) describes his concept of phenomenology of the social world as being the study of lived experience from the unique perspective of the individual engaged in the experience. Benner (1985) considers the phenomenological approach as being of great use to health care research; she states, 'No laws, structures, or mechanisms offer higher explanatory principles'. I believe that the use of this technique can provide a deeper understanding of how individuals in counselling perceive their role in the process and may give insights into ways that they may change as a result of the counselling process. The thoughts and feelings of the co-researchers (research participants) at a particular time are unique, and circumstances affecting the respondents will never be exactly the same again. It can therefore be argued that anything said on a specific day can only be viewed as being relevant at that time. There will, however, be much information and material recorded that will provide meaningful and useful research matter and enhance insight into the way the respondents view and experience the caring process.

I believe that it is the holistic nature of this type of research that is its strength. Chinn (1985) supports this view and points out that quantitative research has weaknesses that are the real strengths of qualitative research. Tatano Beck (1994) believes that, following years of logical positivism dominating health care, a philosophy that is congruent with the holistic and interactive characteristic of caring relationships is required. She offers phenomenology as providing a 'better fit' conceptually with health care relationships. A qualitative methodology allow people to explore each other, takes into consideration their very humanity and acknowledges all influences, allowing the 'specialness' of the individual to be revealed and interpreted. Hermeneutic phenomenology offers a potential framework to guide the researcher through the process of understanding the expressed experiences of individuals. This can lead to a deeper and clearer understanding of the effectiveness of counselling.

## Phenomenological methodology in nursing research

There is a growing tradition towards the use of phenomenology in nursing research. Several studies will be considered as they show the power of this approach to enquiry. All of the studies at some stage allude to the inadequacies of positivist research methodology when exploring the areas of their individual studies and specific research questions. As mentioned above, it is essential that the methodology chosen matches the question asked (Field and Morse 1985, Cormack 1991, Stevens et al. 1993, Parahoo 1997). Subjects for phenomenological research that support its use in this type of study have included:

*Caring for a patient: a phenomenological enquiry* (Thibodeau 1993): This study explores the lived experience of caring for a parent. Thibodeau states that it is genuine understanding of a situation, not the categorization of that situation that is of importance to nursing. In her study, she interviewed family members and used a multicase, comparative, situational analysis design. Ten family units were selected for inclusion; emic (individual perceptions of the experience) descriptions were juxtaposed with etic (other people's perceptions of the experience) descriptions. The experiences of caring for a parent can be extremely difficult to explore. Those family members who had few demands on time, space and energy perceived the experience of caring for a parent as a positive experience. However, members of some other families described negative emotions. Her research findings revealed important information that had implications to help nurses and social workers to care better and to provide focused resources for social assistance. The findings could also add to the debate surrounding health policy at a central level with many elderly parents being cared for at home by their children at a much-reduced cost to the taxpayer.

*Nurse-teachers' attitudes to research* (Bassett 1994): In this study, I explore the perceptions of nurse-teachers relating to research education for student nurses. Using phenomenology as the research methodology, I was able to explore the controversial and often intensely difficult issues surrounding the personal abilities and attitudes of the teachers towards practice-based research education. The study revealed a great deal of insight into the changes in nurse education and how they were dealt with by those effected by the move from hospital-based to university-based education.

*Critical care nurses: ethical dilemmas – a phenomenological perspective* (Bassett 1995): In this study, I was able to help reveal some of the extremely personal and complicated ethical dilemmas faced by nurses caring for those patients who are critically ill. Six intensive care nurses were surveyed to explore their beliefs relating to care of critically ill patients. They spoke of issues relating to professional empowerment, feelings of impotence and powerlessness, and a deep desire to care for the patients in a highly focused way.

*A hermeneutic study of the experiences of relatives of critically ill patients* (Walters 1995): In this study, Walters asked 15 female family members of critically ill patients about how it was to see their relative in the intensive care unit. The research participants revealed potent new insights into the lived experiences of family members of critically ill patients. These insights help intensive care nurses to understand the issues and problems faced by visitors.

*A phenomenological study of the nature of empathy* (Ballie 1996): This study explores the perceptions of empathy in nurses from surgical wards. Themes are developed and insights relating to the empathic relationship between patients and nurses are given. A number of interesting areas are identified in the research, such as differences between the literature and the nurses' actual perceptions, the perceived value of life experience of patients and nurses in enhancing understanding. Finally, the study suggests that, to develop empathy, nurses need a natural ability to empathize and also require some experience in both nursing and life.

*Ethical problems in nursing the terminally ill* (Bassett 1996): This study considers the lived experiences of nurses caring for terminally ill patients in a hospice setting. The respondents expressed moving insights into the difficulties of caring for patients in the final stages of life. In doing so, the research provides valuable insights into this stressful care setting enabling nurses and managers of care to explore ways of providing support for nurses in cancer/palliative/terminal care settings.

*Clinical learning experiences and professional nurse caring: a critical phenomenological study of female baccalaureate nursing students* (Kosowski 1995): This phenomenological study analyses and describes how 18 nursing students learnt professional caring during their education process. Highly intuitive aspects of individual nursing experiences were identified by the respondents in this research that has the potential to inform the approaches of teachers, clinical nurses and managers to organizing and enhancing care programmes.

*Using a phenomenological research technique to examine student nurses' understandings of experiential teaching and learning: a critical review of methodological issues* (Green and Holloway 1997): This study examines the respondents' attitudes towards and understanding of the sometimes controversial educational methods relating to experiential teaching and learning. The students voiced clear definitions of what experiential teaching and learning was to them. They expressed the abilities to transfer experiential teaching and learning situations freely to other experiences, both classroom and clinically based.

*Experience of social support in rehabilitation: a phenomenological study* (Natterlund and Ahlstrom 1999): This study explores the experiences of 37 patients suffering from muscular dystrophy. The researchers wanted to understand the issues relating to the social support available to the patients when engaged on a rehabilitation programme. The findings expose the real and personal issues experienced by muscular dystrophy patients. Many important insights were gained that could then be incorporated into future rehabilitation programmes.

This list is certainly not exhaustive, but shows the kinds of issues that have been considered as best suited for phenomenological research methodology.

Phenomenology does not attempt to provide an answer; indeed, there may not be an answer. What it can do, however, is provide a greater level of understanding of those issues. All practitioners need to consider ways of improving their effectiveness to their clients and also need to move towards the ability to prove cost-effectiveness of their services. It is true that other methodologies could be used to explore the above research situations. However, to begin to understand the intensely personal issues surrounding complex subjective occupation, care, and hard-to-penetrate, difficult and inaccessible areas of life, phenomenology has no real methodological rivals. If one truly wishes to understand the phenomenon at hand, phenomenology is a powerful way of exploring intensely personal and hidden aspects of life.

# Nurses' perceptions of care: a phenomenological study

Following on from the previous section, this chapter will now use a study as an example of how this type of research may be used in real practice. This study explores how 15 qualified nurses and six students understand care and caring. It uses phenomenology as its method and describes the emergent themes of the co-researchers using extracts from their interviews. Fifteen categories of meaning are highlighted, which are then collapsed into five themes: 'making a connection', 'encouraging autonomy', 'giving of oneself', 'taking risks' and 'supporting care'. The findings are compared with the literature and implications for practice are made.

## Literature review

The literature review was carried out using the electronic databases 'Cinahl' and 'Medline' using the keywords 'care' and 'caring'. The databases were accessed for the years 1970 to 2001. The citations available in the search were 2,231 articles that matched the search criteria. A carefully selected sample covering nurses' perceptions of care are offered below.

## Nurses' perceptions of care and caring

Larson (1986) uses a caring assessment instrument (CARE-Q) to measure oncology nurses' perceptions of what they thought would make the patients feel cared for. The study revealed that it was the expressive humanistic

behaviours that ranked highest, such as listening, comforting and express-
ing sensitivity.

Dyson (1996) carried out a study aimed at eliciting nurses' conceptualizations of caring attitudes; to do this she utilized the repertory grid
technique. This method of inquiry examines the research participants'
own individual perceptions of incidents, events and people. The participants, nine in all, were all hospital nurses. She concludes that caring is a
combination of what the nurse does and what the nurse is. In her research,
significant themes emerged, these include 'consideration and sensitivity',
'honesty and sincerity', 'general approach' and 'giving of oneself'. All of
the above characteristics underline the importance of the humanistic and
psychosocial aspects of care within the caring process. On the question
'What is the nurse like as a person?' strong themes emerged, including consideration and sensitivity, giving of oneself, and the nurse's general
approach. On the question 'What does the nurse do?' work style was considered to be a key component. Important themes emerge, such as having
time for patients, appearing unhurried and being in control.

Coulon et al. (1996) carried out research to explore the meaning of what
'excellence in nursing' meant to nurses themselves. They sent open-ended
questionnaires to students in their first year of study and to registered nurses who had previously graduated from hospital-based nurse-education
programmes: 156 respondents in total. Responses revealed that at all times
the patient was at the centre of the nurses' concern. This concern was
grounded in professional practice, delivered both competently and in
holistic care for the patients and their families.

Rittman et al. (1997) asked oncology nurses what skills and attributes
they used in caring for their patients. Data collection consisted of narratives written by six nurses – all with at least five years of oncology nursing
experience. They were asked to write about an experience that taught them
something about what it means to care for a dying patient. Themes were
taken from the narratives and were interpreted in the following ways:

- knowing the patient and the stage of illness
- preserving hope
- providing for privacy

The cornerstone for oncology nursing was considered to be the provision of privacy while dying.

McQueen (1997) explores the verbalized experiences of 12 nurses relating to the care they provided for their patients. Following analysis of the
data, the following themes were identified as being of relevance to care:

- direct patient care
- caring for patients having a pregnancy terminated

- caring for patients having a miscarriage and problems with fertility
- caring for terminally ill patients
- caring for patients who are emotionally upset
- caring for patients behind a façade
- caring for relatives
- caring for the nurse

In summary, the nurses, in describing their work in great detail, highlighted the importance to them of a high level of interpersonal and humanistic care for the patients in their workplace.

Critical-care nurses were included in a study by Bush and Barr (1997), in which 15 nurses were asked to describe their lived experiences of caring. Caring in the critical-care area was revealed to be 'a multidimensional, complex process involving assessing and addressing patients' and their families' unique needs with the goal of improving the patients' condition, and acknowledging nurses' living out of caring ways in their own lives'. Four categories were drawn from the research. These were:

- nurses' feelings
- nurses' knowledge and competence
- nurses' actions
- patient and family outcomes, and nursing rewards

For the 15 nurses involved in the exploration of the caring activities in their daily work, caring was seen as a series of processes consisting of an affective process, a cognitive process, an action process and an outcome process.

## Methodology

As with any inquiry, it is the way that the exploration is undertaken which is the key to its success or otherwise (Field and Morse 1985, Cormack 1991, Stevens et al. 1993, Parahoo 1997). This study uses phenomenology, which uses the lived and expressed experiences of the nurses themselves, and it explores the feelings and beliefs of the individuals involved in the caring process.

## Sample

The qualified group of co-researchers comprised 15 nurses working in a variety of posts including psychiatry, theatres, critical care, education, community and management. The group of student co-researchers comprised six members, two from the first year, two from the second and two from the third year of the advanced diploma in nursing studies (ADNS) course.

Semi-structured interviews were carried out lasting between 30 and 50 minutes; they were tape-recorded and later transcribed. All participants gave informed consent to the research.

## Using the data

The process of interpretation used Colaizzi's (1978) approach to phenomenological analysis. All of the transcriptions were read to develop a feeling for them and to make sense of them. The taped interview was listened to, and on the transcript a code letter and number were inserted. This code highlighted that there was in the transcript a word or phrase that had significant meaning. Codes were added as necessary throughout the taped transcripts. Statements and phrases directly relating to the caring experience were carefully highlighted in the margins and designated into textual units.

Significant statements that pertained to the phenomenon of care and caring were collected. Statements were then organized into categories in relation to perceived meanings. At this point, the transcripts had been read numerous times and the tape recordings were reviewed to hear the co-researchers' tone of voice. Research field notes were compared to the other data sources to ensure accuracy. The meaning of each statement was then spelt out; this is known as formulating meanings. At this stage, it was important to see beyond what was actually said to make inferences about what was meant or implied. The formulated meanings were then arranged into categories 15 categories of meaning.

- making contact
- encouraging autonomy
- tuning in
- using skills and knowledge
- hands on
- getting involved
- physical and emotional
- taking risks
- getting a buzz
- being there
- challenge
- giving of oneself
- caring for colleagues
- commitment and ideals
- humour

These categories were then collapsed into five themes to expedite the process of writing up: 'making a connection', 'encouraging autonomy', 'giving of oneself', 'taking risks' and 'supporting care'. Again, at this stage, the transcripts were reviewed to ensure that the new thematic cataloguing fitted with the co-researchers' meanings.

The themes are briefly presented in the following section, with selected extracts of the transcripts.

## Making a connection

There can be little doubt that creating a relationship between the nurse and the patient is essential for effective nursing care to take place.

### Tuning in

It may be that a sign of an effective nurse is the ability to cut to the chase, as it were, and rapidly assess the patient and help them cope with their illness or operation.

> **Chris**: How might you define caring?
>
> **Lynn** (day surgery): To sort of tune in. What I'm trying to say is that you might do something out of your own needs to care for somebody without actually defining what they want. So maybe it's a reciprocal understanding that you are not doing things for somebody else, because you need to care for them or it might be that you do something or care about somebody else in a way that you want to be cared for, but in fact it's not. It's about knowing what other people want and then responding to that.

### Learning to make a connection

The students in the sample were all highly motivated and enthusiastic about their training and the experiences they were gaining. The students were, even early in their training, already picking up on the ways they might make effective connections.

> **Chris**: Could you name, say, the four characteristics that might make someone a good nurse?
>
> **Alice** (second-year student nurse): Good communication skills. Being able to listen and interpret, not just verbally but body language and, you know, using that ... I think you need to be intuitive, because ... you do pick up on things that people don't say or that other people outside might see it. ... It's like fitting a jigsaw together: you might pick up on one thing and somebody else might mention it and you think, 'Well, yeah, that fits.'

Making a connection with the patients was seen as being important to the nurses. They saw it as a vital factor in the effectiveness of the caring relationship.

**Encouraging autonomy**

The notion of the 'empowerment in patient care' is an issue that also seems to be important to the nurses in this study.

> **Anne (theatre):** I'd say it's definitely about providing the patient with something, but it's also about empowering that patient where possible.

Anne seemed to want to ease the patients' fear and anxiety by rendering them more autonomous and giving them more control over their care.

> **Jill (theatre):** To give the patients real independence and control of their own care, which is what modern nursing is about rather than doing everything for them, then you have to do a certain amount of teaching of patients in terms of health promotion, health education and in some cases teaching how to actually give physical care, like for someone with diabetes how to give their injections.

Cathy, amongst other aspects of care, saw the encouragement of patient autonomy as being important in her care:

> **Cathy (psychiatry):** I'm quite interested in all the issues around what empathy really is and actually being able to demonstrate it and how patients perceive that and as part of that actually being able to empower people, because, obviously, if you work in psychiatry, you are dealing with a fairly downtrodden group of people in our society; so it's also really important to be able to make people have control and not feel controlled and have choice and not feel as though choices are being made for them and be able to influence what happens to them and what happens in the service that they are part of, and things like that.

Cathy links empathy with empowerment here. She also seems to have a strongly developed sense of justice and sees her patients sometimes as being very much at the powerless end of the spectrum. Like their more experienced colleagues, students saw empowerment as an important way to underpin the care they gave.

*Learning to empower*

The significance of empowerment is seen in the responses of Alice, who had this to say:

> **Chris:** In what ways do you care for your patients?
>
> **Alice (second-year student nurse):** And being able to get alongside that . . . and maybe try and help them through that, to be a guide and kind of be part

of the process, to make decisions. You may not have a totally positive outcome, but you may be able to help somebody live with the situation.

Alice, even with patients who are dying, saw empowerment as being a very real way to care for her patients.

There are real indications that nurses do see the greater provision of patient autonomy as a positive part of caring.

## Giving of oneself

Caring, it can be argued, is the essence of giving of oneself. Nurses give to patients, of this there can be little doubt, time, energy and effort and they spend time learning the skills and gaining the knowledge both as students new to nursing and also as students learning throughout their nursing career. Jack gave a personal definition of care. He certainly seemed to see it as giving something of himself or giving something up:

> **Jack (teacher)**: I think care is about giving something up. Care is about giving up part of yourself, whatever that might be. It could be time, energy ... which a person either chooses to appreciate or not. So it's giving anything of yourself so that a person can benefit from it.

Cathy, too, described giving something of herself in the way she cared for her patients:

> **Cathy (psychiatry)**: It's just I find it really rewarding to work with people where you are having to give of yourself an awful lot.

### Learning to give of oneself

The students who were interviewed, in similar ways to the other themes, again seemed to be picking up the importance of ways of caring from the experienced nurses that they had worked with on the wards. They identified the importance of caring for the patient in both physical and emotional ways similarly to the experienced nurses.

> **Carl (first-year student)**: Well, care I think is a whole range of things really, but I mean if ... you want to kind of try and put it in a nutshell, I think caring is basically identifying what ... people's needs really are, and that's not only the physical need ... it's all sorts of different other needs: I suppose psychological and emotional needs as well.

Carl seemed to be strongly influenced by more experienced nurses, he went on to point out:

**Carl**: But it's his or her ability [the nurse's] as people to relate to someone with a medical or psychological need.

Role-modelling seemed to be an important aspect of the ways that students learnt to care for patients.

## Taking risks

Taking risks in nursing is not about putting patients at risk by acting in any kind of cavalier fashion; instead, the term was associated with pushing the boundaries of accepted care outwards.

Jack seemed to believe that nurses who truly cared sometimes took risks in providing care.

> **Jack (teacher)**: Because, if you are really delivering care, then you are not worried about what you do. It's like if you go on a course and you are not telling the truth then it's going to trip you up. In practice if you are really caring then perhaps no one is going to trip you up about it. People recognize that you are caring, but when you actually get back to it, you know, she gives herself, she stops afterwards, she never has a break, you know, you really think she is a caring person, but when it comes down to it, will I get a complaint or will I get anything said against me? Or this might go to court and you think, 'Oh she's not caring.' It's a form of self-protection and she's thinking about herself and not her patients.

The above account indicates that an element of courage is required to care for one's patient in a more radical way. The courageous nurse is the one who, in order to care fully, in the nurses' view, meets the patient in what some nurses might consider to be a deeper way.

I asked Cathy to describe a caring situation from her practice.

> **Cathy (psychiatry)**: I remember being in the situation where I was in a human sense dealing with this lady who was really high and unable to concentrate and all those other problems, and her communication was a bit disrupted, but [she] was really saying, 'I don't need that injection. I don't want it. I just need not to drink, calm down and keep taking the lithium.' I ended up refusing to give the injection against the psychiatrist's wishes and this went on for a number of weeks, and there were some really difficult issues around stopping the other nurses giving the injections.

Cathy took a risk in a professional sense in not obeying the doctor's order in giving the injection. It is hard for a nurse to refuse a medical order; however, it is sometimes essential in order to protect the patients from harm.

The extracts above indicate that some nurses feel it necessary to, at times, make a stand against their professional colleagues' interpretations of normal nursing procedures or protocols in the cause of caring.

Students also need to be courageous at times and sometimes to take risks. The student co-researchers also saw the requirement to take risks as being an essential part of caring for patients. In their cases, 'taking risks' meant standing up for their patients when they felt that the care they received was less than they felt the patients deserved.

*Learning to take risks*

Alice had at times stood up for patients when she felt that her patient was not being cared for in the right way:

> **Alice (second-year student nurse):** I think the key to good care is being strong enough to object if you don't agree with something.

Issues relating to the theme taking risks indicate that some of the nurses in this study see that in order to provide a high standard of care they must at times step out of the normal parameters of nursing care. The culture of nursing does tend to be rigid and even constricting in the ways it makes nurses conform to its norms. I believe that nurses do need to push out from the positions of professional safety and to begin to take risks for their patients.

## Supporting care

Here the co-researchers identify the fact that they believe there are certain essential factors required to ensure that care can be delivered effectively.

Anne is a manager in the operating theatres, with responsibility for her team. Anne's priorities for care seem to incorporate a wider, more encompassing view. She feels that to provide good care to the patients her staff members need caring for as well.

> **Chris:** But you are a manager. What about your colleagues?
>
> **Anne:** The first thing from a priority point of view would be the care of the patient, but thereafter my role is definitely to make sure that the staff are OK. That's this old adage of 'Who cares for the carers?' and I don't think a lot of people do, and I don't think we are very good at caring for each other.

Some nurses identify that a major part of their caring role is the creation of a caring environment. Lynn greatly enjoyed the caring one-to-one contact she had with her patients but stated that it was vital to have a system of organization in place to support care.

**Lynn (day surgery):** Dealing with patients, that's obviously the most important part, but what I'm learning more and more is that I love that side of it. I love that contact and I love making patients feel welcome and that they are being looked after properly, but increasingly there's problems with actually getting systems of work in place so that that occurs, and increasingly I'm looking at these important things.

## Summary of the study

This study has allowed the co-researchers to expose some personal conceptualizations of their caring roles as nurses; it has also provided many important insights into some of the ways in which they provide care for their patients. In addition to this, the study has also provided views of the rich contextual fabric that forms each co-researcher's nursing life.

### Limitations of this study

The expressed experiences, as recorded and interpreted in this study, of each nurse are only applicable to them at the time of the interview, and as such can only provide further limited, though valuable, understanding of their views of what care might be to them. Nurses are not all the same in the ways in which they care for their patients: they reflect the patients' changing needs for different types and intensities of care by giving them different types and intensities of care. These differences in care requirement and care provision depend upon the context.

### Comparison of the findings with the literature

The emergent themes are generally represented in the literature. The findings and expressed beliefs of the co-researchers do appear to underline and reinforce the very complex nature of the phenomenon that we call care.

### Aspects of making a connection

The expressed feelings, attitudes and beliefs described ways of caring that epitomize the perceived closeness which was deemed essential by the co-researchers when caring for their patients. The theme was strongly linked to the nurses' ability to listen, comfort and express their sensitivity to the patient. Many studies found these aspects of care important to both patients and nurses (Rieman 1986, Taylor 1993, Morse 1994, Coulon et al. 1996, Dyson 1996, Leinonen et al. 1996, Rittman et al. 1997, McQueen 1997, Halldorsottir and Hamrin 1997, Kralik et al. 1997).

## Aspects of encouraging autonomy

The section entitled 'encouraging autonomy' considered the notion of 'empowerment in patient care' as perceived by the co-researchers. It was seen as an issue of importance to the nurses in this study. It was the only theme that did not contain subcategories, suggesting perhaps its strength as a value for nurses. References to empowerment appeared in the following literature: Morse (1994), Hankela and Kiikkala (1996), Halldorsottir and Hamrin (1997) and Barr and Bush (1998).

## Aspects of giving of oneself

Caring is the essence of giving of oneself. Nurses give time, energy, effort, they spend time learning the skills and gaining the knowledge both as students new to nursing and also as students learning throughout their nursing career. To simply provide mechanical care may not be enough in their eyes; providing care without genuineness was not seen as adequately caring for their patient. Again, the literature supported the findings of this study: Jensen (1993), Hughes (1995), Dyson (1996), Vincent et al. (1996), Bush and Barr (1997), Halldorsottir and Hamrin (1997), Staden (1998), Wolf et al. (1998) and Radwin (2000).

## Aspects of taking risks

Taking risks in nursing was associated with pushing back the boundaries of accepted care. It was about moving from the defined boundaries of the profession and developing new and innovative ways of caring for patients. Again, the literature identified this concept as being a real one, though it was referred to in only one paper: Vincent et al.'s (1996) study.

## Congruence of findings to the literature

There are strands throughout the literature that do link strongly with the views and attitudes as expressed by the co-researchers in the study. In terms of the themes 'making a connection', 'encouraging autonomy' and 'giving of oneself', there is a strong correlation between the expressed words of the co-researchers and the literature. That is to say that the findings have a close match with other recent and influential studies on the ways that nurses and patients see caring. This is also true of the nurses in my study, as their expressed views seem to mirror the previous studies in several important ways. This would lead me to recommend that nurses need to be cautious about implementing strategies of care which they feel will enhance the patient's experience. Before they implement anything, nurses need to be quite happy that the patients want them implemented. This makes clear the need for more research into the relationship between nurses' perceptions of what 'good' care is, and patients' perceptions of what they see as 'good' care. This study only considers the views of a small section of nurses and nurse students, which do little to indicate what patients may need or want.

Moving on to consider the other emergent themes 'taking risks' and 'supporting care', their presence in the literature is much less well represented. It is here I feel that new insights into these notions are to be found in the present study. My own view is that nurses do need to innovate and implement change in their practice. However, there is associated with this trend risk: the risk of stepping from the norm, the risk of challenging other more dominant health care professional groups, the obvious one perhaps being medicine, and also challenging managers and even academics; this needs considerable courage and strength from nurses wishing to make changes.

Supporting care would seem to be associated with nurses who have developed a more managerial or organizational role within the caring environment. The issues surrounding the need for effective management systems that streamline communication and decision-making are clearly expressed in the views of some of the co-researchers. Leading on from this, and in fact closely related to it, both the experienced nurses and the students place the value on psychosocial support. Commitment and ideals are again considered as important to nursing though are rarely mentioned by many of the co-researchers (that is not say the other co-researchers do not have commitment and strongly developed ideals); when referred to, however, they were seen as very important but could lead to some frustration if other members of the team did not share them to the same degree.

### Implications for practice

As stated above, this research is qualitative and is not expected or able to provide us with absolute truths about care, caring and the ways that nurses understand and provide that care. It is therefore only possible to provide greater understanding and insight into what it is to care as a nurse or student nurse, which I feel this study has achieved. Having said that, by transmitting the findings in various ways to the wider audience, there may result some changes in individual practice from those who might read the study's findings. Nursing is an important part of the health care system in all parts of the world. What this study has shown, albeit in a limited way, is some of the ways that nurses feel about caring for their patients. They speak of the ways that they strive to make connections with the patient and of being there for them. They speak of encouraging greater independence in their patients, enabling a deeper involvement in the caring process with patients and their families becoming full partners in care. They speak of the giving of something of themselves to the patients in order that the patients can receive the incredible benefits from the nurses' skills and knowledge. They describe the ways that they put themselves on the line and take risks to improve the services which they can provide for the patients. Finally, the students in particular describe the emotional pressure and pain that they feel in caring for the patients. All of these factors showing, I believe, the great value nurses and nursing have to the patients in need of timely and high expert nursing care.

**Implications for education**

This research has implications to educators of nursing. The main issues, as I see them, are related to the identification of care as being at the centre of the curriculum. Care, I believe, has tended to be pushed from that position by various forces in recent years. It is important to re-affirm care as the central and unifying tenet of nursing. It really does need to be placed centre stage not just by merely being constantly referred to in lectures but also by the identification of the need for real support for practitioners of nursing and students alike. Teachers need to remember what it was like to begin to learn to nurse and in doing so help students to cope better with the emotional assaults that can occur in nursing.

# Conclusion

This study has provided insights into nurses' conceptualizations of what they see their own nursing care being. I feel that, if this group is representative of other British nurses and students, I have real faith that nursing care is alive and well in Britain and has a bright future too. It is important for policy makers at all levels to accept that nurses want to care for the patients. In order to do this, the Government, educationalists and managers and nurses themselves need to put the structures into place that will enable this to happen. This is needed for the sake of the patients of which, after all, any of us has the potential to become.

# References

Ballie L (1996) A phenomenological study of the nature of empathy. Journal of Advanced Nursing 24(3): 1300-1308.
Barr W, Bush H (1998) Four factors of nurse caring in the ICU. Dimensions of Critical Care Nursing 17(4): 215-223.

Bassett C (1994) Nurse teachers' attitudes to research: a phenomenological study. Journal of Advanced Nursing 19(3): 585-592.

Bassett C (1995) Critical care nurses: ethical dilemmas – a phenomenological perspective. Care of the Critically Ill 11(4): 166-169.

Bassett C (1996) Ethical problems in nursing the terminally ill. European Journal of Palliative Care 2(4): 166-168.

Benner P (1985) Quality of life: a phenomenological perspective on explanation, prediction and understanding in nursing. Advances in Nursing 8(1): 1-14.

Bush H, Barr W (1997) Critical care nurses' lived perceptions of caring. Heart and Lung: The Journal of Acute and Critical Care 26(5): 387-398.

Chinn P (1985) Debunking myths in nursing theory and practice. Image 17(2): 45-49.

Cohen MZ (1987) An historical overview of the phenomenologic movement. Image 19(1): 31-34.

Colaizzi PF (1978) Psychological research as the phenomenologist views it. In Valle R, King M (eds.) Existential-phenomenological Alternatives for Psychology. New York: Oxford University Press.

Cormack DFS (1991) The Research Process in Nursing. Oxford: Blackwell Science.

Coulon L, Mok M, Krause K et al. (1996) The pursuit of excellence in nursing care: what does it mean? Journal of Advanced Nursing 24(7): 817-826.

Drew N (1989) The interviewer experience as data in phenomenological research. Western Journal of Nursing Research 11(4): 431-439.

Dyson J (1996) Nurses' conceptualisations of caring attitudes and behaviours. Journal of Advanced Nursing 23(8): 1263-1269.

Field PA, Morse JM (1985) Nursing Research: the application of qualitative approaches. Beckenham, Kent: Croom Helm.

Gadamer H (1989) Truth and method. In Weinsheimer J, Marshall DG (trans., eds.) Truth and Method. New York: Crossroad.

Green S, Holloway G (1997) Student nurses understandings of experiential teaching and learning: a critical review of methodological issues. Journal of Advanced Nursing 30(5): 1215-1227.

Halldorsottir S, Hamrin E (1997) Caring and uncaring encounters within nursing and health care from the patient's perspective. Cancer Nursing 20(2): 120-128.

Hankela S, Kiikkala I (1996) Intraoperative nursing care as experienced by surgical patients. AORN 63(2): 435-442.

Hughes L (1995) Teaching caring to students. Nurse Educator 20(3): 3-5.

Jensen K (1993) Care: beyond virtue and command. Health Care for Women International 14(4): 345-354.

Knaack P (1984) Phenomenological research. Western Journal of Nursing Research 6(1): 107-114.

Kosowski MMR (1995) Clinical learning experiences and professional nurse caring: a critical phenomenological study of female baccalaureate nursing students. Journal of Nurse Education 34(5): 235-242.

Kralik D, Koch T, Wotton K (1997) Engagement and detachment: understanding patients' experiences with nursing. Journal of Advanced Nursing 26(3): 399-407.

Larson PJ (1986) Cancer nurses' perceptions of caring. Cancer Nursing 9(2): 86-91.

Leinonen T, Leino-Kilpi H, Katajisto J (1996) The quality of intraoperative nursing care: the patient's perspective. Journal of Advanced Nursing 24(8): 843-852.

McQueen A (1997) The emotional work of caring, with a focus on gynaecological nursing. Journal of Clinical Nursing 6(3): 233-240.

Morse JM (1994) Comfort: refocusing of nursing care. Clinical Nursing Research 1(1): 91-113.

Moustakas C (1994) Phenomenological Research Methods. Thousand Oaks, Ca: Sage.

Natterlund B, Ahlstrom G (1999) Experience of social support in rehabilitation: a phenomenological study. Journal of Advanced Nursing 30(6): 1332-1340.

Oiler C (1982) The phenomenological approach in nursing research. Nursing Research 31(3): 178-180.

Omery A (1983) Phenomenology: a method for nursing research. Aspen: Advances in Nursing Science.

Parahoo K (1997) Nursing Research Principles, Process and Issues. London: Macmillan.

Radwin L (2000) Oncology patients' perceptions of quality nursing care. Research in Nursing and Health 23(3): 179-191.

Ray M (1994) The richness of phenomenology, philosophic, theoretic, and methodologic concerns. In Morse JM (ed.) Critical Issues in Qualitative Research. Thousand Oaks, Ca: Sage.

Reinharz S (1983) Phenomenology as a dynamic process. Phenomenology and Pedagogy 1(1): 77-79.

Rieman JD (1986) Non-caring and caring in the clinical setting: patients' descriptions. Topics in Clinical Nursing 8(2): 30-36.

Rittman M, Paige P, Rivera J et al. (1997) Phenomenological study of nurses caring for dying patients. Cancer Nursing 20(2): 115-119.

Roche M (1973) Phenomenology, Language and the Social Sciences. Boston, Mass: Routledge.

Schutz A (1967) The Phenomenology of the Social World. Chicago, Ill: Northwestern Press.

Spiegelberg H (1960) The Phenomenological Movement: a historical introduction. The Hague: Martinus Nijhoff.

Staden H (1998) Alertness to the needs of others: a study of the emotional labour of care. Journal of Advanced Nursing 27(12): 147-156.

Stevens P, Schade A, Chalk B et al. (1993) Understanding Research. Edinburgh: Campion.

Tatano Beck C (1994) Phenomenology: its use in nursing research. International Journal of Nursing Studies 312(6): 499-510.

Taylor B (1993) Ordinariness in nursing: a study. Nursing Standard 7(29): 35-40.

Thibodeau J (1993) Caring for a patient: a phenomenological enquiry. Nursing Outlook 14(1): 15-19.

Vincent J, Alexander J, Money B et al. (1996) How parents describe caring behaviours of nurses in paediatric intensive care. American Journal of Maternal/Child Nursing 4(5): 197-201.

Walters AJ (1995) A hermeneutic study of the experiences of relatives of critically ill patients. Journal of Advanced Nursing 22(9): 998-1005.

Wolf Z, Colahan M, Costello A et al. (1998) Relationship between nurse caring and patient satisfaction. Medsurg Nursing 7(2): 99-105.

# CHAPTER EIGHT

# Historical analysis

JUDY REDMAN

## Introduction

During the short period that I have been preparing this chapter, the *Guardian* has carried an editorial explaining that history as an academic subject is endangered, and the *International History of Nursing Journal* has ceased publication. The British Prime Minister's prediction that history would judge (and presumably acquit) him over the UK Government's intervention in the invasion of Iraq in the spring of 2003 led to the *Guardian's* gloomy observation, but the *IHNJ's* demise is of more immediate concern to anyone who wishes to undertake historical research in nursing. The first is likely to turn out to be a premature obituary – the second could be an early indicator that support for historians of nursing may be becoming harder to obtain at a time when there is a future-orientation to the gathering of the evidence base for clinical practice.

Articles published in North America during the early 1990s tell of the lack of both practical support or serious professional regard for nurses studying history during the previous two decades (Sarnecky 1990). Since then, though, there has been a flourishing of interest in the history of nursing and midwifery in the USA and UK, as seen in the highly successful triennial History of Nursing conferences held in various cities around the UK, the establishment of the UK centre for nursing history at Queen Margaret University College, Edinburgh, which also runs a postgraduate diploma programme in the history of nursing, and regular seminars held by history of nursing colloquia around the UK.

So what is the appeal of history when the *IHNJ's* editor had earlier commented that:

> To some hostile critics, studying and writing about the history of nursing is a harmless if dull way of filling empty hours. Health care's equivalent of trainspotting (Sarnecky 1990).

178

To me, history is not just a grim amorphous past that is entirely separate from what I do now and what I see when I look out of the office window but an essential dimension to contemporary nursing practice. On the other hand, it is not a series of entertaining tableaux to be viewed in isolation from each other. Trying to find a definition of what history is can be tricky, however. In general, books about history avoid giving a simple definition of what it is or warn the reader that the simple definition is inadequate. As a nurse, I found that this had a familiar echo in questions about what nursing is and what kind of research nurses should be engaged in. To a large extent, working out what I understood 'doing history' involves and which perspective(s) I should take in interpreting those aspects of the history of nursing and health care I am studying has been as much a part of undertaking historical research as answering the research questions I set out with. I have become aware that the way in which the past is (re)presented by historians has led to heated debate among professional historians.

## Historical research

My experience of historical research originated in a long-term interest in the workings of the NHS as an undergraduate student and then as a nurse. After ten years of nursing, I completed a masters degree in Health Services Studies, during which I wrote my dissertation on the effects of competitive tendering in the NHS on staff in NHS laundries during the first round of tendering during the mid-1980s. The subject occurred to me when someone working as a manager in a laundry claimed that one needle carelessly left in a linen skip could potentially lead to the closure of the laundry and the loss of all jobs for what was already the lowest-paid group of employees in the NHS.

I was particularly interested in how policy decisions made in the centre of government affected people working at the point in the hierarchy that is most distant from where the policy makers were. I was also interested in the extent to which policy makers' intentions may be realized or frustrated at the point of implementation. Finally, I was also interested in how far and in what ways the NHS affected individuals' experiences and expectations of health care, starting from its implementation with effect from 5 July 1948, and with reference to people in daily contact with general hospitals, whether as patients or as people working in the new service. This gave me the starting point from which I could begin the research process. This chapter offers a reflection on what this has involved and in some respects why and how I have revised my original intentions.

# Getting started – some practicalities

As a postgraduate research student, I have found that it is invaluable to obtain expert guidance throughout the research process, which as a complete novice was essential in the early stages. For me, that support came in several guises. First, I was able to discuss my ideas with a professional historian who specialized in the study of the social history of medicine. Although I was not able to begin my research for a further two years because of changed personal and work circumstances, the opportunity to sound out my ideas before I made a firm commitment to undertaking postgraduate research was very helpful. During that conversation, a potential supervisor was recommended to me, and I was subsequently able to register as a postgraduate research student under that person's supervision. Secondly, what were very general ideas were taken seriously and at the same time I was challenged to start clarifying them. Finally, I was given a very useful list of books and articles that would give me an introduction to the social history of medicine and health care.

Once I had registered as a research student, I was required to attend a two-semester module in historiography, which comprised weekly meetings during which all members of the small student group were normally required to participate in analysis and discussion of the work of a diverse range of historians. This facilitated critical exploration of different approaches to the study of history and insight into some of the controversies in the discipline over the nature of history and historical research. The opportunity to undertake a similar unit of study is one that I recommend to anyone embarking on historical research. It should be very helpful for any nurse who is interested in using historical methods in research, particularly if the study of history is unfamiliar.

Thirdly, while this is not something that all those undertaking research for a higher degree can count on, the support of my employers has been very valuable in allowing me to find some time for data-collection analysis and writing my thesis. I have been lucky in securing time for study as part of my professional development during the week, although even with this I have needed to work on my thesis in the evenings and at weekends. Therefore, the final, though not least-important, source of support has been the willingness of my family to put up with my sneaking off to the study instead of going to the park with them.

# Getting on with the research

In any research study, whether for a higher degree or otherwise, there are constraints on what can be done. For me, the main constraint has been time; because of the need to work to pay the bills, I have had to fit my study around the demands of my job and the needs of my family, rather than being able to concentrate on it without interruption from other demands. I was not realistically in a position to travel far from home or spend much time away, as I had young children. I knew that some trips would be feasible but could not build my plans around extended absences. Therefore, I decided that the focus of my study would be the hospitals in one city local to where I live and work. The data I would be using had therefore to be available locally or within easy travelling distance.

While there are a variety of frameworks available, historical research involves systematically locating, interrogating and interpreting data in order to present a new understanding of events in the past and why and how change has taken place in society. This goes beyond the rehearsal of a series of dates and events, which may admittedly be intrinsically interesting but is ultimately unsatisfactory as history because it lacks both context and any sense of the ways in which aspects of human society both undergo change and yet endure. The first step, therefore, was to read the general literature on the topics in which I was interested and gain an understanding of the main events that had taken place. In addition, reading the literature, including studies done by other researchers, helped me to understand that the history of the NHS has controversial elements. Also, it enabled me to refine my research questions further.

Since the late 1950s, a number of studies have been published that offer analysis of the origins and early development of the NHS (Eckstein 1958, Willcocks 1967, Pater 1981, Webster 1988, Powell 1997, Rivett 1998), while Ham (1981) draws attention to the difference between national policy intention and local implementation reality in his history of the Leeds Regional Hospital Board. The impact of the NHS on the nursing profession at the national level has been the subject of one doctoral thesis and subsequent publications (White 1982), while others have researched different aspects of the profession of nursing in England, through research into the politics of nursing knowledge, nursing's political leadership and the militarization of nursing during part of the period 1948 to 1974 (Rafferty 1996, Scott 1995, Starns 2000 respectively).

# Increasing the body of knowledge

I anticipated that my research would contribute to this body of knowledge by evaluating hospital nursing in the NHS at regional level and by adding further to a still relatively neglected aspect of the social history of the NHS – the contribution of nurses at the regional level to the development of the NHS in its early years and vice versa. I had first to establish the context for the study, and this led me to explore three main areas of literature concerned with the NHS, nursing and the city whose hospitals were to provide my case study.

I first wanted to examine the extent of continuity and change in health care before and after the establishment of the NHS in 1948. Among the issues to consider were the reasons for the development of the NHS into a tripartite structure, which occurred between 1948 and 1974. Controversies in the literature on the issues of pre-NHS financial pressures in the voluntary hospital sector, the contribution of municipal hospitals to the overall provision of facilities and, subsequently, the organization and resourcing of the NHS were also issues that I needed to appreciate.

By this stage, I had decided that the central focus of my research should be on nurses in general hospitals in one English city. I then had to explore the general contextual framework for interpreting the development of hospital-based nursing services in the city, during the first phase of the NHS's existence, between approximately 1948 and 1974. The aim of outlining and examining the policies and statutes that affected the development of general hospital nursing in England was again to encourage an exploration of the relationship between central policy and local reality.

The third aspect of exploring the context of continuity and change in the city's general hospital nursing services involved analysis of the relationship between national policy and local NHS hospital management. I considered what changed and what did not appear immediately to do so in relation to hospital services in the city, before and after the establishment of the NHS.

Although I had identified a general area of interest for my research, I still had to find a clearer focus. Once again, having the opportunity to discuss this with my supervisor at an early stage was essential, although the precise scope of my research could not be entirely clarified at this stage. This was because I had first to identify whether the data existed for research. My general reading identified five themes to be addressed that dealt respectively with nurse recruitment, nurse education, nursing work, nursing management and the changing relationship between hospital and community in the city between 1948 and 1974. I was advised to visit the city archives to find out what was available locally as the next step in the research process. This was done to ascertain whether there was sufficient material to support the research I proposed to undertake. The lack of data is a potential stumbling block, which in my naivety I had not considered at all.

## Documentation and its collection

Identifying the archived documents that I was to use took several months, although this was largely because my survey coincided with a period of maternity leave when I had very few opportunities to visit the local archives and even fewer to use the Internet to search for more distant collections. Perhaps the archivists would not have minded visits by a baby and a toddler, and I have occasionally seen children in the reading room, but I decided not to risk it as the baby was particularly prone to vomiting during the early months of his life, and my toddler was very fond of doing 'art'.

Undertaking research in history through analysis of archived records involved becoming familiar with the concepts of primary and secondary sources. The straightforward way to differentiate between the two is that *primary* sources are ones which are seen in their original form. Primary sources include minutes of meetings, letters, diaries, photographs and other materials, including physical objects. Facsimiles of original documents may also be available, when the original document is very fragile or otherwise difficult to make direct use of. My research involves interpretation of events that took place in the fairly recent past, and the materials I am consulting are generally in quite good condition. Even so, sometimes individual documents have literally been crumbling at the edges or where they have been folded. Also, there are rust marks around staples and paper clips. Archivists are not only skilled in helping you to locate the materials you need to consult, they are also able to show you how to avoid causing any further damage to the documents you do read.

By contrast, *secondary* sources are the works of historians who have read the primary material and are presenting an interpretation of their contents. These may quote passages from the minutes, letters and diaries or reproduce photographs or illustrations of objects, but do so in the context of an analysis of their significance. The general literature I had consulted comprised secondary texts, some of which were based on original research carried out by the author, others representing a survey of existing work.

On the other hand, as most books or articles concerning the study of history point out, the distinction can become blurred. For example, while Maggs' (1983) research for *The Origins of General Nursing* was based partly on nursing records as primary sources, he also read popular novels of the period that he was researching, also as primary sources of information about contemporary, popular views of nurses and nursing. I have myself read nursing textbooks published between the mid-1940s and mid-1970s as primary sources of information about what teachers of nurses at the time recommended to their readers as best nursing practice. This last example may appear strange. After all, the fact that something was recommended in a textbook, even one that appeared in many editions, such as Pearce's *A General Textbook of Nursing*, which was already in its tenth edition in 1949, is not a guarantee that it was observed in clinical practice. However, this does point to the need for historical research to involve more than simply reading and noting the main points in any source. What is also interesting about the textbooks is that the owners have added notes in the margins, and sometimes fuller notes written on loose pieces of notepaper have been left in them. There are several advantages to using archive material, such as committee minutes, not least among these is the intrinsic interest in entries such as the following:

> It was agreed that a dog should not be purchased for Hallwood Hospital, but that the possibility of further domestic assistance be investigated.

In addition, the opportunity to read a first-hand account of an event – and even the opportunity to return repeatedly to interrogate it when a human witness would long since have either died or withdrawn from the process – allows the researcher to interpret and re-interpret as part of an iterative process allowing possible connections between events to be highlighted and tested.

However, the fact that there is no guarantee that a particular archive exists must be one of the greatest potential drawbacks. I had imagined that the NHS must produce vast quantities of paper, just waiting to be tackled by intrepid explorers such as myself. I had worked in five different NHS hospitals and had helped to produce reams of paper records. Not so – the production of the records and their retention are two entirely different matters. While those who work in the NHS are indeed obliged to produce careful records of all aspects of its activities, from the minutes of meetings held to the details of surgical operations, from records of tenders received to supply specific goods and services used in the NHS to nursing care plans, not all of those records can be retained indefinitely, because there is not sufficient storage space in which to keep them. Ham's (1981) introduction to his study of policy making in the NHS in the Leeds region indicated that he had enjoyed access to a wide range of committees' minutes and papers pertaining to administration at all levels within the region he was studying.

However, it was not like this in the region where the hospitals that I wanted to study were located. While material existed, the continuity of individual series of records appeared to be interrupted and the data incomplete, with several years' worth of minutes from one of the major hospitals not having been retained at all. Those records that had survived had been stamped as received in a particular office. It seems possible that one individual – perhaps two – had been responsible for filing them and thus keeping them until the records were passed on to the local archives department. A gap of several years was then followed by a similar run of several years of retained records. Moreover, the records that had survived were largely those of the central committees in the administrative structure, those with policy making or executive responsibilities, and while reference might be made to other reporting committees their records had not necessarily survived. The latter not infrequently included the records of committees that dealt directly with nursing matters.

# The problem of not having enough to go on

This left me facing the possibility that there would not be sufficient data for my research, but two pieces of luck rescued me. The first came in the person of an archivist who was interested in NHS records and who had been working with some material that had been deposited but was not yet listed. This meant that it had not been identified with a unique accession (or reference) number which general readers could use to obtain documents, and so was not listed and described in either the archives' special lists, which alert the researcher to collections on specific topics or in the general indices. The archivist very kindly gave me a copy of an unfinished list of material that included reference to boxes of unsorted material which had been deposited by one of the local hospitals. Because of this, I was able to identify the documents for retrieval to read and make notes on. Some of this material seemed to yield little useable information, although it took a considerable amount of time to survey. I wanted to make more than cursory notes of what was there in case it did turn out to be of use at a later stage. For example, the fortunes of the staff cricket club seemed far from my interest in general hospital nursing but might turn out to be useful in analysing aspects of the hospital's role as an employer, or the relationships between various staff groups working in the hospital during the time that the club existed. More immediately useful was the discovery that the records for several of the 'missing years' were in the unsorted files along with detailed architects' plans for new buildings on the same hospital site.

My second piece of luck came from a chance conversation with a colleague who knew that a former member of staff at another local hospital had saved large quantities of documents which had been destined for destruction. This included a complete set of nursing staff records for one of the hospitals in the city, along with minutes of meetings held on two hospital sites. In addition, there were photographs of members of the nursing staff, many unlabelled, sadly. This collection is now in the local city archive. It is unlisted as yet, though I have been able to access the documents for my research.

Historical research, as is the case with any other kind of research, must be systematically and rigorously conducted. When I began surveying the local archives, I therefore started to keep a detailed list of the documents I found available in the archives, as well as material available in the local studies library and – later – one of the local universities. A published list of archives held locally is available, but I have found this to have limitations, not least because it does not include the unlisted material that I had access to. My own list also had to reflect my research interests and so include more detailed information on some of the documents, and less on others. I divided my list into sections according to where the documents were held, with further subdivisions according to the subject or hospital to which the document referred. I organized the list as a table with three columns originally, for the title, date(s) and accession numbers of the documents respectively. I had to revise this format almost immediately as I wanted to record when I had consulted a document and make a note of my first impressions, whether I had made detailed notes or needed to return later for a more detailed consultation, or include notes of links to other documents in which information about a particular issue was included. My own list now has five columns. The first gives the accession (or reference) number for the individual document, the second a title, which tells me more about the contents of the document, the third the date(s) when or between which the document or its constituent parts were created, the fourth is where I record the date(s) when I have consulted the material and the fifth is for comments.

I have saved the template electronically so that I can update the information as and when new information becomes available or when I reread material and note new links or issues to explore further. I make these notes as I work at the archives and cross-reference these to the more detailed notes I keep as I read each document.

In essence, the list serves two main purposes. The first is that it allows me to plan a systematic course through the material available. The second is to allow me to find my way back to that systematic course if and when I go off at a tangent in pursuit of something interesting along the way. One file of newspaper clippings relating to a local hospital contained details of a particularly nasty murder that had taken place in a house two streets away from where I live – which I found quite frightening until I reminded myself that it had happened nearly 50 years before I read the item. Finally, I keep a diary – essentially an annotated plan – that allows me to cross-reference work in the archives with my reading of secondary literature and newspapers and ephemera kept in the local studies library.

While the newspaper clippings had been collected in a file that was deposited along with others containing the records of committee meetings and working groups from one of the hospitals, they did not constitute a confidential record. Indeed, all the information they contained and more was also to be found on microfilm in the local studies library – along with a huge variety of pamphlets, public notices and other items of immediate and peripheral interest. Many of the records I wanted to use had not been made generally available in the public domain when they were first created and were still subject to statutory and other restrictions on their use. Access to records such as those created by different bodies and institutions within the NHS is governed by statute, in the form of the Public Records Acts of 1958 and 1967. These have been supplemented with further guidance in the form of policy statements on general access to public records and specifically on the retention of NHS records.

In essence, these documents are usually available for consultation after 30 years, although this period may be varied either to allow earlier access or to lengthen the closure period. For example, in my own list of archived documents I have noted restrictions on three different registers of nursing staff in the city where I am doing my research. In one case, the files appear to be closed for 26 years from the date of the last record in the file, whereas, in the other two cases, the closure period is 76 years. The reason for this discrepancy is not obvious. Patients' records though are closed for much longer – 100 years, assuming that they survive at all as the article by Higgs and Melling (1997) explains.

NHS records, whether administrative or clinical, may provide only some of the material to be consulted. Records of other bodies, such as trades unions and professional associations, societies, clubs and personal papers may be available, although not necessarily easily accessible. Restrictions on access to these may be imposed by the body or individual that deposits them in the archive, whether this is the Public Record Office, a local record office, archive, university or other institution or learned society. Whatever the reason for the restriction, permission has to be sought to gain access to closed records. If this is forthcoming, it may be that the research can only be conducted within specified limits on the use of the material.

A further limitation on access could be the geographical location of the records. For example, although I identified locally available sources of information for my research, I also travelled to the Public Record Office at Kew, London, to consult the General Nursing Council for England and Wales' records of inspections of hospitals with nurse-training schools. I was fortunate in having a choice of places to stay from which to visit the PRO, but even so the cost of travel was quite high and I used holiday time to make the visits. The Royal College of Nursing's archive is in Edinburgh, and other collections pertinent to the study of the history of nursing are held in various locations including universities or research institutes around the country. Using locally available sources of information has made access easier for me and provides much of the data I require, but it has not been sufficient to support my research into all aspects of my study.

## Using the archives

Archive materials exist for many reasons but generally not with the researcher in mind. So, while I needed to have a clear idea of what I wanted to find out, I also had an open mind about the material I would use in order to interpret the data. In addition, it has been necessary to review and reinterpret the data continually as I have gone along. In this sense, data collection, interpretation of the data and writing have all been taking place simultaneously, and revision of earlier drafts has been necessary throughout the process.

It would be impractical to keep all artefacts generated by human beings – and the archivist is therefore trained not only to keep but also to cull material. The decisions made are framed by legislation but in the context of the perceived significance of specific items. Thus, records of some aspects of the life of an organization may be referred to in the minutes of central policy committees, but the original documents themselves may no longer exist if the subcommittee to which they refer does not meet the criteria for retention. Related to this is the fact that records of even the central committees may be incomplete: even if there is a requirement to retain certain documents by law, the implementation of that requirement may be inconsistent and the actual practice can appear to depend on the motivation of an individual. The significance of specific items may not be appreciated at the time when the process of archiving them takes place – which could in itself be a reflection of the historical context in which archivists work and the changing status of particular occupational groups, such as nursing.

Another dimension that I have experienced is that an archive may be 'complete' in as much as minutes of all the meetings that took place during the lifespan of the committee have survived. However, the depth and range of material contained in a set of minutes can vary, and over time the richness of the account may alter and even fade. The reasons for this can be speculated upon, though it may not be possible to verify them. Perhaps the changes in the nature of the records kept indicate that there was a change in the guidelines under which a record of the minutes of meetings were kept, or a change in the person of the minutes secretary. Alternatively, perhaps it is a reflection of the growing familiarity of members of the committee with each other. Records of meetings held early in the life of a committee or working party may be more detailed if they reflect the need of the various members of that group to inform themselves and each other of the scope and extent of their business and provide details that they would not be able to discover by other means. Gradually, the same people would establish a shared knowledge about their work in the committee and the minutes would only need to mention an issue briefly in order to update members of the committee on what was happening. Also, or alternatively, the different people represented on the committee might establish informal networks of communication that they would make use of to discuss business in between meetings, and these could occasionally or eventually consistently bypass the formal meetings.

In an article published in 1996, the nurse historian Rafferty notes that an important feature of historical research is the lack of control the historian has over the data. Some of the implications of this for the role of the researcher in interpreting the data have been noted above. In addition,

specific archives have been established to collect material on certain subjects, and these may be far from the researcher's base for example, while
some material relating to a specific person, event or organization/institu-
tion may be scattered between several different places. My research
involves the use of archives, while others researching the history of nursing
have been using oral history. In either case, there may be limited opportunities to seek corroboration of the data.

This leads on to a further point, concerning external and internal criticism of the documentary sources. External criticism concerns the
establishment of authenticity of a document. The first aspect to consider is
that the document or artefact may not be genuine. While it is possible that,
as a result of human error, an item could be presented as something it is
not, a document, on the other hand, could be a deliberate forgery –
whether produced at the time the putative document was created and
therefore during the period that is being researched or at a later date.
There are ways in which authenticity can be checked. For example, objective laboratory tests can be carried out to establish whether the paper and
inks used in producing a particular document are ones that were in use at
the supposed time of production. Internal criticism of documents is done
in order to assess whether or not it can be accepted as providing reliable
witness to events. For example, the language used in the document and references within it should not be anachronistic.

Even if it is not a forgery, it could be that the author has either con-
sciously or inadvertently distorted the account of events. Minutes of
meetings within a structure such as the NHS seem unlikely to be forged, and
the normal procedure of meetings in commencing business with a reading
of the previous meeting's minutes and agreement on their authenticity
and/or corrections to be made is one approach to preventing distortion
that takes place as the record is made. However, it is conceivable that pressure to be seen to be producing particular results may lead to deliberately
false records being made, as one high-profile case involving an NHS hospital in the north of England in 2003, where attainment of Government-set
objectives was allegedly considerably embellished, illustrates. Therefore,
even when there does not appear to be a high risk of documents being
forged or inaccurate, there is still a need to seek corroboration of the
records by examination of other sources to establish whether the information in the original can be accepted as factual, probable or possible.

# Reading through the literature

A reading of both the secondary sources and a detailed reading and interpretation of archived material indicated that my research should analyse

the relationship between national and local aspects of the recruitment and retention of nurses, their initial and postgraduate (post-registration) training, the work they did, intraprofessional relationships, including the management of nursing and nurses, and the relationship between the hospital and the community it served. This would allow me to compare the relationship between national policies and local interpretations of these in the context of specific circumstances and facilitate an analysis of continuity and change in each over the period I was studying.

The establishment of the NHS in July 1948 was a major political victory for Aneurin Bevan. In persuading recalcitrant members of the medical profession to participate in the provision of hospital, general practitioner and community health services, he overcame a highly visible barrier to the establishment and success of the new service. However, Bevan recognized that, while winning his battles with the British Medical Association and the medical Royal Colleges was essential to the immediate survival of the new service, without enough nurses to provide patients with day-to-day care, the universal hospital service could not be delivered.

Concerns over the interrelated problems of nurse recruitment and retention predated the NHS's establishment. Furthermore, as therapeutic interventions became more complex, the need for a range of specialized carers grew. During the first 26 years of the NHS's existence, organizational change was paralleled, and even overtaken, by medico-scientific developments. As this happened, the capacity of the NHS to provide a universal and comprehensive range of health services required the availability of not only a numerically adequate nursing workforce but an increasingly diversified and highly technically skilled one.

The leaders of the nursing profession may not have expressed the strong political objections of their medical colleagues to the new services, although some expressed reservations about the state control of hospitals. However, the problem of recruitment and retention of sufficient nurses presented a continuing challenge to politicians as well as to hospital administrators.

I therefore wanted to examine how national policy and local circumstances influenced specific strategies in the different general hospitals of the city and analyse the factors that influenced nurse staffing levels and approaches to the determination of nursing establishments in the hospitals, from the inception of the NHS in 1948 until its reorganization in 1974. I wanted to find out whether local hospital authorities experienced fluctuations in the availability of new recruits and, if so, how they dealt with them. At the national level, there appeared to be increasing requirements for nurses and at the same time widening alternative opportunities for young women seeking work. However, it was also necessary to examine whether the general national picture applied to the local employment opportunities for women.

# Contentious issues

The determination of ideal nursing-staff establishments was both technically and politically contentious. Hospitals were working within limited budgets, and accounts of attempts to change the skill mix and the number of nursing staff in the city's hospitals provide interesting insights into the relationship between people working at different levels within the hospital service. Further questions arise, such as were the hospital authorities successful in their recruitment and retention of staff on a consistent basis, and how did their success or otherwise affect their ability to provide a service to patients? Dilution of the nursing workforce, with non-nursing staff taking on nursing duties, was another strategy, which could be employed to ensure that the service could continue to deliver nursing care, but another question to ask was whether this was done, and what effect either using or rejecting this strategy might have had.

In interpreting the data on each aspect of nursing, there have been a number of questions to ask. For example, given the central importance of nurse recruitment and retention to several official and semi-official reports published in the years leading up to the establishment of the NHS, one question that I have explored is whether and how the relationship between nurses, at all levels, and their employers and the development of recruitment and retention strategies in the NHS differed from those used before. At what stage did those changes occur and why? What was the nature of the process itself and the influences on that process? *The Majority Report* of the Wood Committee (DoH 1947) notes that the terms and conditions under which nurses were employed were unnecessarily restrictive and contributed considerably to attrition rates of over 50% of students from many schools of nursing. However, the quarter of a century covered by the study encompasses a period that is popularly supposed to have witnessed the creation of the teenager, the questioning of the Establishment and the so-called 'second wave' of feminism. Could nursing as an occupation that relied on a constant influx of young women be impervious to these wider, social changes?

The situation of nurses as workers can be traced through nursing staff records where these exist, and, for the hospitals I am studying, these do exist. The information available includes details of changes in terms and conditions of service, career patterns and some insight into the reasons people gave for leaving nursing. This is similar in scope to that which Maggs (1983) used in his study of general nurses at the end of the nineteenth and beginning of the twentieth centuries. The implementation of specific national policy directives related to nursing recruitment and retention, at a local level, can also be examined through the minutes of hospitals' and health authorities' administrative committees.

# Learning the lessons

Having examined the recruitment of staff-nurse training and education, the context of changes in the nature of health services provided by the NHS was the next aspect of the study to be analysed in depth. This aspect of the history of nursing is closely related to general recruitment and retention issues, since the majority of members of the nursing workforce at the time were recruited as probationers, or students, and thus the ability to maintain approval as a training school for nurses, and to attract students, was of central importance.

During the period of the study, the major proportion of the nursing workforce comprised unqualified nursing staff, without whom the work of the hospitals would have been compromised. Between 1948 and 1974, however, the structure of this unqualified part of the nursing workforce nationally changed. For example, problems in recruiting students produced responses that included greater use being made of unqualified staff in non-training posts, the identification of non-nursing duties to be devolved to other grades of hospital staff and more flexible attitudes to conditions of service for all nursing grades. In addition, the establishment of pre-nursing courses in collaboration with the local education authority and interagency co-operation in the development of hospital-careers information for schools were pursued. The records provide data that allow for the characteristics of the nursing workforce to be explored, including demographic trends and senior nurses' perceptions of what constituted acceptable and unacceptable levels of ability and behaviour in students and their junior colleagues. Demographic data include information on students' previous work and educational experience, age on joining the hospital, religion, gender and marital status. Patterns of training can be discerned from information about the range and duration of ward and department placements attended by students. Subjective information on the performance of students, and non-training employees, is also available. In addition, the inclusion of all grades of nursing staff in the records of the Royal Hospital means that changes in the relative proportions of trained, training and non-trained nursing grades over time can be traced.

While much of the material for this chapter relates to the pre-registration training of nurses, the development of what were termed 'postgraduate' courses for nurses will also be analysed. These followed, largely, acute medical and surgical specialities. Again, these courses appear to have served more than one purpose, both enhancing the skills of nursing staff working in these areas of the hospital and providing recruitment opportunities for the hospital.

Having considered the training of staff, I wanted also to consider what those staff actually did in their day-to-day nursing work. Therefore, I revisited my data in order to answer questions about the nature of nursing work, and how this was affected by the new arrangements for health care delivery in the hospital setting. This is a topic that has received relatively little attention in the literature, although Rivett's (1998) history marking the first half-century of the NHS does include a very useful and well-contextualized account of the development of clinical nursing work, as opposed to nursing administration or education. It is a subject that can be approached from different directions. First of all, the interdependence of hospital medical and nursing work should be considered in relation to the development of medical and surgical specialization between 1948 and 1974. The *Hospital Surveys*, published in 1945, summarized the strengths and shortcomings of the hospital services of the early 1940s, including inadequate accommodation, poorly situated and uncoordinated services, with duplication in some areas and absence of essential services in others. The *Surveys* also noted the unplanned and patchy development of consultant and specialist services in English health services prior to the foundation of the NHS.

In January 1948, the Ministry of Health issued a memorandum to regional hospital boards, later developed for publication as a pamphlet in 1950, which set out brief guidelines on the strategic planning of consultant services in a wide range of medical and surgical specialities. A closely related aspect of this chapter will thus comprise a consideration of developments in therapeutic interventions between 1948 and 1974 and an examination of the extent to which developing specialization in hospital care affected global and specific requirements for nurses. It will also consider the extent to which hospital authorities were able to meet these requirements.

Medical specialization and therapeutic developments brought with them an increasing demand for more qualified and specialized nursing staff in specific parts of the general hospital, such as the operating theatres, the intensive care unit and the neurosurgical unit.

Thirdly, during the period under study, attempts were being made at the national level to define the scope of nursing practice and the differences between 'nursing' and 'non-nursing' work. The Wood Committee (DoH 1947) had divided on precisely this issue, Cohen's *Minority Report* (Cohen 1948) being premised on the argument that the NHS's numerical requirements for nurses could not be determined until the nature of the nursing work required had been defined. The Nuffield Provincial Hospital Trust conducted a job analysis of hospital nurses, published in 1953, which was debated by the Standing Nursing and Midwifery Advisory Committee between 1953 and 1961. In addition, the Ministry of Health's Standing Nursing and Midwifery Advisory Committee produced guidance on specific nursing procedures and the organization of care between 1949 and 1971. Again, in what ways these discussions were developed at local level, and with what impact, is an issue for consideration.

The next theme for exploration was the relationships between nurses at different levels in the hospitals, and between nurses and others working in the hospital. Having addressed the recruitment and training of nurses, and the nature of the work for which they were prepared, the next step therefore is to consider the management of nursing work and conditions of work. This is an issue that has been identified clearly as of central importance in studies of the relationships between national health policy and politics and general nursing. Changes in the managerial role of nurses have to be seen in the context of more general changes in the status of all nurses. In turn, analysis of this aspect of the organization of the hospital necessitates examination of interprofessional relationships.

Over the period under study, nurses were largely excluded from membership of the administrative committees, which ran the hospitals, although senior nurses did attend meetings of those committees, which dealt directly with nursing matters. As Scott (1995) notes in her study of nursing at the Ministry of Health, it was only in 1968, when the Salmon Committee's recommendations on the senior nursing staff structure were accepted, that the management of nursing changed and senior nurses were enabled to form the nursing committees that would determine nursing policy.

This aspect of the research is still being undertaken and examines the extent to which nurses were able to influence the operation of the hospitals where they worked. It will also examine the extent to which senior nurses were able to influence the conditions of work of nurses, including the weekly hours and shift patterns that nurses worked. In addition, it will examine the attitudes of nursing leaders in the various hospitals to auxiliary grades, including enrolled assistant nurses, and how these altered over time – particularly in response to recruitment crises.

Finally, I shall return to the issue that first intrigued me, namely in what ways and how did the advent of the NHS affect the relationships between the hospitals and the local community. In 1948, the new NHS hospital administration inherited much that had existed in the administrative structures which had preceded it, particularly where the former voluntary hospitals were concerned. People who had run the hospitals before 1948 were often members of the new committees, and the freedom to determine the precise nature of the committee structures initially led to the retention of familiar administrative structures.

However, as the NHS developed, tensions became increasingly apparent in the tripartite structure where Ministry of Health policy limited the freedom of the periphery to determine its own administrative structures. In addition, longer-serving members of committees and boards gradually retired or died in office and were replaced by people who had not been immersed in the culture of the voluntary or municipal hospitals. Towards the end of the period of the study, for example, adoption of the Salmon

Committee's recommendations was followed by changes in the involvement of senior nursing staff on the committees of the hospitals.

Additionally, hospital administration became increasingly professionalized, reflecting the more complex nature of the NHS. While there continued to be a role for lay people in the NHS, this was less one of controlling than of monitoring the work of the health and hospital authorities. These developments give rise to two main questions. First, 'In what manner and degree did interprofessional relationships develop during the period 1948 to 1974?' and, secondly, 'To what extent, if any, did the existence of the NHS shape health politics at the local level?' Prior to the establishment of the NHS, and during its early years, the membership of the hospital committees was primarily composed of members of the local community. The funding of the city's hospitals before the NHS was established reflected a strong local involvement in the voluntary hospitals, and the municipal hospitals were also, by virtue of their funding by the rate-payers, 'owned' by the local community. Funding of the hospitals in the NHS was not only more remotely organized at the national level but control over where funds were spent, even in the case of the teaching hospitals, was no longer in the hands of the local committees to the extent that it had been before 1948. In what manner and to what extent did connections between the city and its hospitals develop following the establishment of the NHS from 1948 until 1974?

What started as a general idea and vaguely defined questions has thus developed into much more coherent work.

## Summing it all up

From very early in the research process, I have been expected to write chapters for my thesis – albeit in draft. I have also to identify and discuss the strengths and weaknesses both of my arguments and the way in which I write and so learn to become my own critic. While this was by no means an easy skill to develop, it has been very useful, allowing me to clarify my thoughts and intentions as well as improving my written style. Initially, I was met with the assessment of my first piece of work as 'not history – but policy', which I found completely bewildering as I had written an account of something that had happened in the past, using a range of appropriate sources, and expected this to be sufficient. So the experience of undertaking historical research has helped me to become more critical in my thinking and as a reader of material I encounter in my working and non-working life.

In addition, there are two other benefits that I can immediately point to. First of all, I had become used to skim-reading information, only picking up the useful bits. Using historical research has helped me to speed up my reading – but has also made me read the whole document or record so that I can appreciate the full context of the information I am seeking. It has also given reading whole books back to me – which I always enjoyed before busy-ness got me out of the habit. Secondly, in order to read, I have to use public transport as I can only find time to read on the bus. So we have given up one of the family cars – who would have predicted that the study of history could be environmentally friendly?

> Unquestionably, research is the key to a better future for nursing. The discipline urgently needs more studies undertaken from a wider variety of approaches to answer the many grave questions confronting it today ... All methodologies, including historiography, should be accorded equal respect and support by all members of the discipline of nursing (Sarnecky 1990).

# References

Cohen J (1948) A General Textbook of Nursing: a comprehensive guide (tenth edition). London: Faber & Faber.

Department of Health (DoH) (1947) The Wood Committee. Working party on the recruitment and training of nurses. London: HMSO.

Eckstein H (1958) The English Health Service. Cambridge, Mass: Harvard University Press.

Ham C (1981) Policy-making in the National Health Service. London: Macmillan.

Higgs E, Melling J (1997) Chasing the ambulance: the emerging crisis in the preservation of modern health records. Social History of Medicine 10(1): 127-136.

Maggs CJ (1983) The Origins of General Nursing. London: Croom Helm.

Nuffield Provincial Hospitals Trust (1953) The work of nurses in hospital wards: report of a job analysis. London: NPHT.

Pater JE (1981) The Making of the National Health Service. London: King Edward's Hospital Fund for London.

Powell MA (1997) Evaluating the National Health Service. Buckingham: Open University Press.

Rafferty AM (1996) The Politics of Nursing Knowledge. London: Routledge.

Rivett G (1998) From Cradle to Grave: fifty years of the NHS. London: King Edward's Hospital Fund for London.

Sarnecky MT (1990) Historiography: a legitimate research methodology for nursing. Advances in Nursing Science 12(4): 1-10.

Scott EJ (1995) The influence of the staff of the Ministry of Health on policies for nursing 1919-1968. DX192212 London, University of London (PhD thesis).

Starns P (2000) March of the Matrons: military influence on the British civilian nursing profession 1939-1969. Peterborough: DSM.

Webster C (1988) The National Health Service Since the War: volume 1. London: HMSO.

White R (1982) The Effects of the National Health Service on the Nursing Profession 1948-1961. Manchester: University of Manchester (PhD thesis).

Willcocks AJ (1967) The Creation of the National Health Service. London: Routledge and Kegan Paul.

# Index

access issues
  action research, 40–41
  ethnography, 119–120
  historical analysis, 186–187
  illuminative case studies, 100–101
action research, 30–32, 45–47, 48–50
  clinical governance in infection
    control, 52–54
  defining an ICU-acquired infection, 37
  experiences from the general adult
    ICU, 40–45
  experiences from the paediatric ICU,
    38–40
  hygiene compliance, 52
  objective measurement of patient
    outcome, 37
  parameters, 32–33
  pilot and control wards, 33–34
  practical applications, 51–52
  researcher's experiences, 47–48
  staging site-specific infection, 37
  two areas, 36–37
  valid research, influencing nurses to
    use, 34–36
*ad hoc* observation
  ethnography, 132
  focus groups compared with, 11–12
  illuminative case studies, 100
  *see also* participant observation
Ahlstrom, G., 162
aims of research
  ethnography, 122
  grounded theory, 60–61
alternative explanations, grounded
  theory, 84–85

anonymity, *see* confidentiality issues
archives, historical analysis, 182–184, 185,
  187–189
axial coding, 67, 75–78
audience for research
  ethnography, 120
  focus groups, 21
audiotapes, *see* tape recordings
authenticity of historical documents, 189

Ballie, L., 162
Bassett, C., 161, 162
Bassey, M., 128
best fit, notion of, 84, 85
Bevan, Aneurin, 190
bias issues
  focus groups, 8, 9
  grounded theory, 57, 58
  literature reviews, 57, 58, 91
  illuminative case studies, 91
Brentano, Franz, 156

caring relationships between nurses and
  patients, phenomenology, 154,
    163–165, 175
  data analysis, 166–167
  encouraging autonomy, 168–169,
    173–174
  findings, 172–175
  giving of oneself, 169–170, 173–174
  implications for education, 175
  implications for practice, 174–175
  limitations of study, 172
  literature review, 163, 172, 173–174
  making a connection, 167, 172, 173–174

197

Printed in the United Kingdom
by Lightning Source UK Ltd.
119371UK00001B/85

9 781861 564405